Fit & Pregnant

The Pregnant Woman's Guide To Exercise

Fit & Pregnant

The Pregnant Woman's Guide To Exercise

by

Joan Marie Butler, RNC, CNM

VITESSE PRESS

Montpelier, Vermont

Fit & Pregnant
The Pregnant Woman's Guide To Exercise

Published by Vitesse Press
PMB 367, 45 State Street
Montpelier, VT 05601-2100
www.vitessepress.com

Library of Congress Cataloging-in-Publication Data

Butler, Joan Marie, 1953-
  Fit & pregnant : the pregnant woman's guide to exercise / Joan Marie Butler. -- 2nd ed.
      p. cm.
  Includes bibliographical references and index.
  ISBN-13: 978-0-941950-40-4
  1. Pregnant women--Health and hygiene. 2. Exercise for women. 3. Physical fitness for women. I. Title. II. Title: Fit and pregnant.
  RG558.7.B88 2006
  618.2'44--dc22
                    2006024224

Photo credits: Josh Hanford pages 103, 115; Suzanne Beste pages 105, 163, 175; Mary A. Mansfield page 153; Tom Thurston pages 138, 171; Dick Mansfield pages 121, 169; Dawn & Tim Allen page 116; Joan Marie Butler all other photographs.

Cover and book design by RavenMark, Inc.
Manufactured in the United States of America

10 9 8 7 6 5 4 3 2 1

Distributed in the United States by Alan C. Hood, Inc. (717-267-0867)

For sales inquiries and special prices for bulk quantities, contact Vitesse Press at 802-229-4243 or write to the address above.

Contents

Foreword

Pregnancy is a time of both profound transition and great opportunity. As your body changes and you move forward toward motherhood, or mothering an expanded family, the most important thing to remember is this: while pregnant, the only way to take care of the baby is to take care of yourself. This is a wonderful time to "clean up your act" by improving your diet, developing stress reduction strategies, and exercising regularly.

Exercise is an integral part of the lives of many women I see in my practice. I encourage women to exercise throughout their pregnancies. For already active women, I ask the specifics of what they do, and it is rare that I feel the need to curtail anyone's program. Usually the opposite is true. I advise a minimum of thirty minutes of cardio, four times a week, and state that forty-five minutes five times a week is optimal. If they are already doing more I do not discourage it, though I do recommend a rest/cool down for those doing vigorous cardio exercises for more than forty-five minute intervals. I recommend that women listen carefully to their bodies and if their activity is causing them pain, they should modify what they are doing.

Fit and Pregnant outlines many popular physical activities and provides advice on how the reader can safely continue to exercise during and after pregnancy. The examples from women all over the country are particularly interesting and emphasize that each woman has different experiences with exercise in pregnancy.

I like the new chapter incorporating Pilates and yoga. I believe yoga is fabulous for pregnant women, not only because it increases strength and flexibility during pregnancy, but also teaches skills that can be used in labor, specifically how to use your mind and breathing to release into sensations in your body. The final chapter is one of the most valuable in the book. With the current epidemic of childhood obesity, all new families need to be aware of the risks of a sedentary childhood. Too much screen time coupled with too little outdoor play has ramifications beyond the obvious physical ones. Integrating your fitness activities into family fun is one of the greatest gifts you can give your children.

Fit and Pregnant is realistic about the benefits of exercise. I tell my patients that in addition to the mental benefits of getting out and exercising, they will have fewer aches and pains in the third trimester, a quicker recovery after birth, potential prevention of pregnancy problems, moderation of weight gain, and a higher level of confidence in their physical abilities and more physical stamina, both of which help make labor shorter and more endurable.

Joan Butler takes a realistic approach to integrating exercise into your life both during pregnancy and afterwards. Her decades of experience and personal commitment to physical fitness are reflected in this very readable and informative book.

Laurie Foster, CNM, CPM, MS
Laurie and her husband live in Vermont and have raised three children in an active lifestyle. Presently one is a ski racer, another a track athlete, and the third a ski instructor/surfer/soccer player.

Introduction

I wrote the first edition of *Fit & Pregnant* shortly after giving birth to my son. In the ten years since, he and his sister have grown into young athletes as I have continued to work with hundreds of pregnant women each year. Though little has changed in the basic research regarding exercise and pregnancy, the concept is now widely accepted such that exercise is part of the prescription for a healthy pregnancy. Today, many forms of exercise offer specific routines tailored to pregnant women. The updated version of this book takes a look at some of these practices, including Pilates, yoga, and using an exercise ball – all popular for their accessibility and health benefits.

Fit & Pregnant is for active women who want to become pregnant – or are pregnant. Women swell the ranks of walkers, cyclists, cross country skiers, and runners and are responsible for much of the growth of activities such as aerobics, in-line skating, kayaking, and mountain biking. Some work out to control weight or to tone up; others do it just for recreation. Many female athletes, from seven to seventy, train daily for competition in their chosen sport.

Do you fit into one of these exercise categories? If so, you are one of the women to whom this book is addressed – women who are physically fit and athletic, and quite often wondering, along with their partners, just how to safely stay fit while pregnant.

Prior to the 1980s, physicians usually advised pregnant women to rest and avoid heavy exertion. In 1985, the American College of Obstetricians and Gynecologists (ACOG) established general guidelines for exercise during pregnancy. These guidelines were very broad and not applicable to the very fit woman. Fortunately, new guidelines released in 1994 and updated in 2002 now call for a more personalized approach to designing an exercise program. Each pregnancy is special and each exercise program will be unique. You should work closely with your nurse-midwife or physician in personalizing your own program to be Fit and Pregnant.

As a certified nurse-midwife and athletic woman, I am frequently asked about exercise and pregnancy. Patients, and their partners, are eager to work toward a healthy pregnancy and delivery. I find that many women share the common goal of staying fit during pregnancy and reaping the physiological as well as the psychological benefits of an exercise program.

I wrote this book to help women, at all levels of fitness, design a personal exercise program for their pregnancies. I look at pregnancy from the vantage point of the fit woman and start by discussing the effects of exercise on fertility. Then, I outline some of the physiological changes you can expect, review some of the basic exercise guidelines, and discuss nutrition. One of the features that has made *Fit & Pregnant* popular is the woman-to-woman advice and sharing of personal experiences from world-class athletes to recreational exercisers. We will look together at a number of exercise activities that women engage in to stay fit during pregnancy. For each activity, I discuss some of the special body changes that occur during the course of a normal pregnancy. Finally, I cover postpartum exercise and how you and your newly expanded family can stay fit.

The material and guidance I share with you is based on my research and knowledge on the topic and my twenty-five years of working with pregnant women. My own exercise program before, during, and after pregnancy, gave me insight and inspiration as did the experiences of other active women we interviewed.

This new book would not have happened without the help of many. Heidi Hill, a young mother of two (and a runner/skier), did much of the book's revising and gathered new pregnancy stories. Laurie Foster, an experienced midwife who has attended over 1000 births, wrote the preface and provided a sharp technical eye on the manuscript. Dick Mansfield, the publisher, planted the idea for this book with me many years ago and has been instrumental in getting this new edition into print.

But the book would not be what it is without the personal stories of fit women, who had varied results in their exercising through pregnancy programs who were willing to share those experiences, good and not so good, with us. Their stories are wonderful reading and enrich the book. Reading these stories will hopefully inspire you to create your own fitness program over the next nine months – for your own health and the health of your baby.

Joan Butler, RNC, CNM

Chapter 1

Exercise and Fertility

S ince you are reading this book, I suspect that you are a woman who exercises and are either pregnant, or planning to become pregnant. That's great! As you will see in the chapters ahead, exercise is an important component of a healthy pregnancy. Exercise, at an intense level, however, may affect your ability to conceive. So let's start by discussing menstrual cycles.

Menstrual Cycles

Janet is a mother of four and a runner. Back before her first child, she noticed, while training for a marathon, a change in her menstrual cycles when she increased her running mileage from 25 to 40 to 50 miles a week. Her periods were further apart and she missed one period. Though her weight stayed the same, it took six months for her cycles to return to normal after the marathon. She conceived her first baby four months later. With her subsequent pregnancies, she cut back her mileage during the times she was trying to get pregnant.

Ann, a triathlete, noticed that during the summer months she occasionally missed one or two periods. She spent summers training seriously and raced two or three times a month. Ann is a small, muscular woman whose weight would drop three or four pounds during this time of intense athletic activity. Her cycles were normal during the winter.

To better understand the exercise-related changes in Janet's and Ann's menstrual cycles, let's first take a look at how our reproductive cycles normally work. A normal menstrual cycle is between 20 and 40 days. To determine the interval between your periods, count from the first day of one period to the first day of your next period. If you have a 28-day cycle, the first half of the cycle, days 1 through 14, is called the follicular phase. The second half, days 14 to 28, is the luteal phase.

Your hypothalamus and pituitary glands, located in the brain, send messages through hormones to your ovaries and uterus. The hypothalamus gland signals the

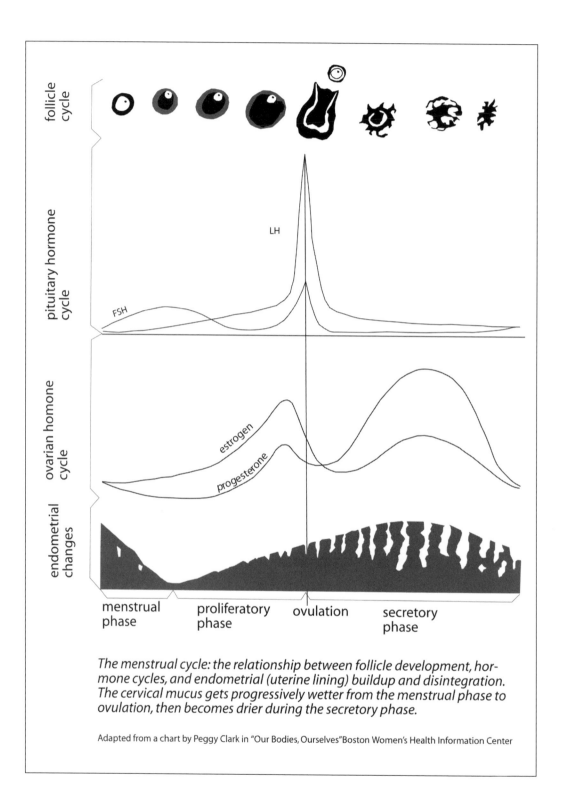

follicle cycle

pituitary hormone cycle

LH

FSH

ovarian homone cycle

estrogen

progesterone

endometrial changes

menstrual phase

proliferatory phase

ovulation

secretory phase

The menstrual cycle: the relationship between follicle development, hormone cycles, and endometrial (uterine lining) buildup and disintegration. The cervical mucus gets progressively wetter from the menstrual phase to ovulation, then becomes drier during the secretory phase.

Adapted from a chart by Peggy Clark in "Our Bodies, Ourselves" Boston Women's Health Information Center pituitary gland to release follicle-stimulating hormone (FSH). In turn, FSH stimulates your ovaries to develop follicles — immature eggs. These follicles then release the hormone estrogen, which causes the lining of the uterus to become thicker in preparation for pregnancy. As the estrogen levels rise, luteinizing hormone (LH) and FSH rise to peak levels. This surge in hormones releases a mature egg from the ovary — causing ovulation. Pregnancy can occur if a sperm joins the egg and fertilization takes place. For the next two weeks, the luteal phase of the cycle, the hormone progesterone further prepares the lining of the uterus for implantation of the fertilized egg. If pregnancy does not occur, then the progesterone level drops and bleeding begins around day 28.

Not all women fit this 28-day cycle, though most have fairly regular menstrual cycles. The interval from menstruation to ovulation can vary, but the time between ovulation and menstruation is the most consistent for all of us and is usually 14 days. It is possible to have a period without ovulation and vice versa, but usually amenorrhea — missing periods — signals a disruption in ovulation. If you are not ovulating, you cannot conceive.

Menstrual Irregularities

Research has helped us to understand some of the effects of exercise on our menstrual cycles, but there is still much that we do not understand. From what we do know, we recognize that there are many causes of irregular cycles. Basically, irregular cycles are due to a disruption in the functioning of the hypothalamus communicating to the pituitary gland, the ovaries, and the uterus. The result may be amenorrhea (absence of menstrual periods), oligomenorrhea (infrequent periods), or a disturbance in the luteal phase of the cycle.

How does exercise affect your menstrual cycles? Let's use running as an example. When you run at high intensity, doing such things as speedwork, competing, running more than 30 miles a week, you cause a rise in beta-endorphins. (Suddenly increasing your mileage can have the same effect.) These "feel good" hormones give you a "runner's high," but they also can suppress the release of gonadotropins (FSH and LH) from the pituitary gland. Similarly, vigorous running releases cortisol from the adrenal glands. High cortisol levels also interfere with the release of FSH and LH. When this happens, ovulation does not occur and menstruation ceases.

Researchers who examined the menstrual cycles of 205 runners found that elite runners who ran up to 80 miles a week were at greatest risk for developing amenorrhea. The runners who developed amenorrhea had lower levels of estrogen and a drop in their bone density. Low estrogen levels, which also occur in menopause, put these runners at risk for stress fractures and osteoporosis.

Body fat and body weight also play a role in menstrual irregularities but perhaps not as significant as we once thought. Our bodies need a certain percentage of body fat to maintain our reproductive cycles and ultimately to support pregnancy and lactation. If we reduce these energy stores, we can in turn disrupt our menstrual cycles. Athletic amenorrhea is more common in individual competitive sports like running, gymnastics, ballet and figure skating where a slim body is desirable. Pressure to excel plus the emphasis on low body weight can put these women at risk.

Besides body fat and the physical stress of exercise, psychological stress seems to play a role in menstrual irregularities. Under stress, the adrenal glands release cortisol, which, as mentioned above, is known to interfere with the release of FSH and LH. A classic study in the mid-60s examined young American women who went to live in Israel for a year. Twenty-two percent of them temporarily stopped menstruating while abroad. These women had higher cortisol levels probably due to the stress and anxiety of being away from home and living in a foreign country. Vigorous or competitive exercise can be psychologically stressful for some athletic women and also elevate cortisol levels. It seems that this biological response to stress prepares the body for challenge and directs energy away from reproduction.

"Female Athletic Triad"

"Female athletic triad" refers to the relationship of three medical disorders — disordered eating, amenorrhea, and osteoporosis. Research has examined the prevalence and potential risks associated with these collective disorders. The term "triad" means that the three problems are often seen together and are related.

As noted before, competitive female athletes, especially runners, gymnasts, ballet dancers, and figure skaters feel pressure to maintain a certain body weight for esthetics and improved performance. This "striving for thinness" may lead to food restrictions, fasting, binging, or purging. The extreme end of this is *anorexia nervosa* when body weight drops below 15 percent of normal. *Bulimia* is characterized by recurring episodes of binge eating followed by purging (induced vomiting, laxative abuse or excessive exercise). Reduced body weight or fat can lead to *amenorrhea,* or *oligomenorrhea* (infrequent periods) or luteal phase defects. As mentioned previously, luteal phase suppression occurs when there is inadequate progesterone in the second half of your menstrual cycle. These athletes place themselves at particular risk for the athletic triad.

Low levels of the reproductive hormones estrogen and progesterone can cause osteoporosis, which results in premature bone loss and inadequate bone formation. We usually gain our peak bone mass by age eighteen. For the next twelve years or so, we have the potential to gain bone mass. Studies have shown that some young athletes with amenorrhea may have decreased bone mineral density and thus are at greater risk for stress fractures and premature osteoporotic fractures.

It is not clear just how prevalent the athletic triad may be among female athletes as athletes affected by this problem may deny or hide the symptoms. Additionally, study results are quite varied with some research showing low occurrences for disordered eating patterns or amenorrhea in female athletes while other studies indicate high percentages. There is no evidence to show what the incidence of osteoporosis may be. In any case, treatment for the problem of female athletic triad may require medical, psychological, and nutritional intervention. Prevention and education are also important. Females in "at risk" sports need to develop safe training techniques as well as positive and realistic body images.

If you are trying to conceive, take a look at your current exercise program. What are your fitness goals? How often are you exercising and at what intensity? Are you training for competition or exercising for fun and fitness? Your fitness program should include aerobic activity (running, cycling, aerobics class, walking) for at least 20 minutes 3 to 5 times a week. Concentrate on building muscle strength, aerobic endurance, and overall stamina. Blend weight-bearing activities like running and aerobics with non-impact sports (swimming, cycling). If you are out of shape, begin with low impact sports and start slowly. Walking is a great "first step" to build a fitness program around.

Too Much Of A Good Thing?

There is no specific amount of weight loss, body fat percentage, exercise or stress level that will cause menstrual changes for all women. For example, Roxanne is a runner who averages forty miles a week. While training for marathons, she increases this to sixty to seventy miles. Normally her menstrual cycles are twenty-eight days apart but during the marathon season they are every 22 to 23 days. In contrast, Gail and Alisa, both competitive runners, average eighty to one hundred miles a week and have regular menstrual cycles. In fact, Alisa, whose body fat is approximately 9 percent, (most women average 22 percent) conceived shortly after a vigorous racing season.

Remember, each of us reacts differently to emotional stress. Stress is a part of everyday life, but how we cope is individual. What is stressful to one person may not cause the same reaction in someone else. Our own biology, personality, and experience seem to dictate how vulnerable we are to stress. It is good for each of us to periodically take a look at how we handle stress in our life. The demands of parenting will certainly introduce you to all kinds of new sources of stress. If you find yourself "addicted" to exercise, you need to weigh how much exercise actually reduces stress and how much the compulsion to exercise puts more pressure on you. It is important to find that comfortable middle ground where you reap the rewards, both physical and psychological, of an exercise program but are not driven solely by the goals of exercise.

Can I Get Pregnant?

If you are missing periods, it is likely that you are not ovulating and will not be able to get pregnant. It is important that the underlying cause of your amenorrhea be determined by a gynecological exam and special tests. You can usually reverse infertility caused by exercise once you cut back on the duration or intensity of your exercise program or, if you are too thin, by gaining weight. If you need to gain weight, now is a good time to improve your eating habits and adopt a healthy diet that is rich in calcium before conception. (See Chapter 4) Depending on your clinical evaluation, you may need to take hormones to stimulate ovulation.

Consider visiting your health care provider for a complete physical and health assessment before trying to get pregnant. If you are a competitive athlete you need to discuss how your pregnancy plans will fit into your "off season" of training. Discuss your obstetric and medical history as well as diet and exercise program. Talk about your lifestyle, the work you do, and the type of environment you live in (urban, rural, etc.).

Start thinking about the type of practitioner from whom you would like to receive your maternity care. You have many options including certified nurse-midwives, certified professional midwives, family practitioners, or obstetricians. It is important to find a practitioner who is knowledgeable about exercise during pregnancy.

Consider your choices for place of birth. Do you want to use your home, a freestanding birth center, birthing rooms within the hospital, or a hospital labor and delivery room? Be sure to talk to other women about their pregnancy experiences. After considering all these issues, make a decision that fits you and your partner's needs for one of life's most joyous ventures.

What Others Say

"I generally stayed healthy and consumed no alcohol when I was trying to get pregnant.

"I was undergoing infertility treatment, so I moderated my exercise and tried to eat better."

"I was training for a diving competition when I got pregnant on our honeymoon."

"My pregnancy was not planned, so I did not cut back on my training schedule." (A competitive runner with a 5k personal record of 16:07.)

"I wished I had gotten in better shape before pregnancy. I gained 10 pounds over the winter and bad weather forced me to reduce my running."

"I had broken my foot so we decided to have children. I went from peak racing form (5k personal record 15:12) to a foot in a cast and trying to get pregnant. It only took us one month to conceive."

"Both of my pregnancies occurred while running nearly 100 miles a week." (A competitive runner)

"I had a complete physical and started taking vitamins and eliminated all alcohol. We conceived two months later."

"*Exercise helped me during pregnancies to help me feel better about myself. It also helped me to stay with good eating habits. Exercise is ALWAYS a good thing for me mentally...it is my time, and I love to get out and breath and feel the outside air. The riding and other exercise helped me to have a strong and fit body throughout all the pregnancies.*" Cyclist & mother of three

Chapter 2

Your Changing Body

Change is what pregnancy is all about. You will be struck at times during your pregnancy by the dramatic and sometimes overwhelming changes occurring in your body. It can be startling to suddenly look down and see a moving swollen "ball" where there once was a waistline. This kind of change is obvious, but other changes are subtle. Some changes are physical and some are emotional. For some women, pregnancy is a time when they feel their best and have a sense of inner calm and untapped energy. Others, less fortunate, are plagued by persistent nausea, heartburn, or backache. The changes initiated by pregnancy start soon after conception, continue right up to delivery, and call for you to make both mental and physical adaptations.

The first adaptation you'll face is the reality of being pregnant and all that it means. For many, the response to the news of pregnancy, whether it was planned or not, is one of ambivalence. This is quite normal. You will be trying to imagine the journey ahead, the new demands and role changes, and the tremendous physical changes that will occur. Talking about these mixed feelings and honestly accepting the mixture of emotions as "normal" seems to help most women. If you are physically active, your focus may be more on the physical aspects of the pregnancy and on your changing body. Let's look at some of the physical changes you will face.

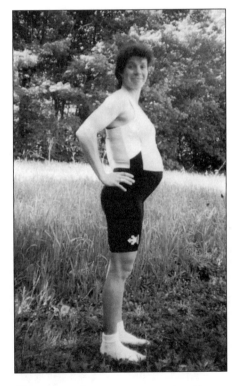

For some women, pregnancy is a time when they feel their best.

Physiological Changes

First Trimester

▶ *Fatigue*

Fatigue is often one of the early signs of pregnancy. If you are used to having a lot of energy and going out and exercising each day, this early sign may surprise you. Fatigue is often described as an all-consuming feeling of being tired and without energy — and it seems to arrive regardless of sleep. A combination of factors, the most important being the tremendous hormone changes you are undergoing and the metabolic demands of the growing fetus, cause fatigue. Try not to let fatigue stop you from exercising — cutting back is fine — but exercising will help metabolize the hormones that cause fatigue. Fresh air and movement often improve nausea as well.

So try to create a balance between exercise and rest. There will be days when your body is telling you to cut back on exercise — so do it. Take short breaks or take an exercise day off to help you get through this phase. Your impulse may be to fight the fatigue and "gut it out" — doing more or forcing yourself to complete a preset goal. But this is the time to listen to your body and realize that by the end of the third month, the veil of fatigue will probably begin to lift.

▶ *Breast Changes*

The hormones of pregnancy, estrogen and progesterone, are responsible for breast changes throughout pregnancy. In the first few months your breasts may be tender and swollen. The nipples may become very sensitive to touch or to the friction from bras or clothing. You can do several things to help alleviate this problem.

Additional breast support, which controls breast motion and allows for evaporation of moisture will help you feel more comfortable. It may also help to avoid synthetic fabrics. If you run or do aerobics, try a supportive cotton bra with wide adjustable straps or a sports bra. One elite runner, during her first pregnancy, told me that she wore two bras for added support. If you are a runner or "stair climber," a temporary change to swimming or cycling — sports which are less jarring — will probably help. Though your breasts continue to enlarge throughout pregnancy, the tenderness tends to abate so you will eventually be able to resume your usual exercises. Later in pregnancy, however, your breasts may begin to leak. The hormone prolactin causes this early milk secretion in preparation for lactation. Wear nursing pads or cut a panty liner to fit the inside of the bra during exercise to solve this problem.

Morning Sickness Prevention

- Eat smaller, more frequent meals
- Eat a few crackers before you get out of bed in the morning
- Get out of bed slowly
- Eat foods high in protein to prevent low blood sugar, which causes nausea. Yogurt, cottage cheese, and milk are good choices for a snack in the middle of the night
- Take your prenatal or multivitamin with a meal or before bed
- Drink fluids between meals instead of with meals
- Avoid foods that are greasy, spicy or fried

Morning Sickness Remedies

- Drink spearmint, raspberry leaf or peppermint tea
- Sip ginger ale or carbonated water at the onset of nausea
- Get fresh air and/or sleep with windows open
- Take deep breaths
- Use TravelBands ™ or BioBands ™ that are applied to the wrist as a form of acupressure to reduce nausea
- Avoid unpleasant odors
- Get plenty of rest

► *Nausea*

"Morning sickness" — waves of queasiness which can hit anytime or any place — is one of the classic trademarks of pregnancy. For me, the smell of sweaty polypropylene clothing would trigger waves of flu-like feelings. I banned my husband's running top from the house for the first three months of my pregnancy. Mary, a competitive cyclist, "never thought (because she is healthy and an athlete) she would feel so ill." Her nausea and dry heaves occurred day and night during her first trimester.

Nausea commonly occurs in over half of all pregnancies. A combination of hormonal changes, a slowed digestive system, the growing uterus, and emotional factors are all causes. The symptoms tend to be worse when your stomach is empty or when you are fatigued, so a key to combating it is to stay nourished and rested.

Nausea may interfere with your desire to exercise. It also may force you to change the timing of your workouts. For example, if you normally exercise at the end of the day when you may be tired and hungry, consider a morning or middle of the day workout. An Olympic champion runner and mother of two said that she avoided nausea by running first thing in the morning and then eating a substantial breakfast. If you are normally an indoor exerciser, try some fresh air — pursuing an outdoor activity such as running, cycling, or skiing may offer some relief from nausea.

Frequent Urination

Early in pregnancy, as the uterus grows, pressure is exerted on the bladder. The need to void often comes during the night (nocturia) or during exercise when you place more pressure on the bladder, especially during running or aerobics. Just plan to empty your bladder before your workout and if needed, during physical activity. Don't, by any means, restrict fluid intake. During your pregnancy, you should drink at least eight glasses of water a day. Hydrate before exercise and keep a water bottle handy. Drinking fluids helps you keep cool during a workout. I recommend that you drink water, but for longer workouts, say over forty-five minutes, you might try one of the healthier sports drinks such as Recharge®.

Second Trimester

During the second trimester (months four, five and six), your body changes will become more apparent. You will feel more comfortable in looser fitting clothing and will want to accommodate your expanding waistline with elastic waistlines or loose oversized shirts. I will discuss specific workout wear for pregnancy and specific sports in future chapters.

► Backache

Low back pain occurs to some extent in most pregnancies. The combination of weight gain and the enlarging uterus alters your center of gravity. You will tend to compensate by drawing your shoulders back and walking with a sway back. This curvature of the lower back is what causes the aching sensation of muscle strain. Women who have relatively strong abdominal muscles are able to give support to the growing uterus and have less muscle strain in the back — so get those abdominals in shape before pregnancy.

Backache can also be a sign of overuse (doing too much exercise) or excessive bending and lifting. Learn how to lift now. Proper body mechanics are important. If you bend at the knees, and not at the waist, and spread your feet apart with one foot slightly in front of the other, you will help save your back. Following pregnancy, when you're lifting a small child and carrying all sorts of baby equipment, you'll be glad that you learned to lift properly.

► Heartburn and Indigestion

The hormones estrogen and progesterone tend to relax the smooth muscle in the gastrointestinal tract, which in turn slows down the digestive process. Bloating and indigestion can develop as food sits in the digestive tract. Some women experience heartburn near the end of the second trimester and into the third trimester. Heartburn, or regurgitation of gastric contents, is caused by a relaxation of the cardiac sphincter of the stomach and displacement and compression of the stomach by the uterus.

► Constipation and Hemorrhoids

As just mentioned, pregnancy hormones, specifically progesterone, slow down the digestive process. The growing uterus causes displacement and compression of the bowel. If you take separate iron supplements for anemia (low iron levels), you may be plagued by constipation. If you had problems with constipation before, pregnancy will increase these problems.

Constipation can cause the development of hemorrhoids. Pressure from the growing uterus and straining when having

Change Your Routine

Kathy, a mother of three, developed varicosities during her third pregnancy. When the varices became uncomfortable during aerobic workouts, she shortened her routine and supplemented it by swimming.

a bowel movement cause dilation of the hemorrhoidal tissue (rectal veins). Diet is an important prevention for both constipation and hemorrhoids. Drinking eight to ten glasses of water a day and eating foods that provide roughage, bulk, and natural fiber is important. Take stool softeners only if advised by your health care provider.

You can relieve the discomfort of hemorrhoids by taking warm tub baths or by applying witch hazel compresses, ice packs, or local analgesic ointments. You can help relieve pressure to the area by lying down with your legs raised. Avoid cycling for long periods or weight training with the Valsalva maneuver (holding your breath and straining) because these activities put more pressure on the dilated veins.

► Ligament and Joint Changes

During pregnancy, the hormone relaxin is being released. Relaxin helps loosen joints and connective tissue to accommodate the growing uterus and to help in delivery through the birth canal. For some women this can be a very subtle change, and for others, the feeling of "shifting bones" in the pelvic region is more dramatic. If you continue to run, you are likely to be more aware of these changes. Your running gait may change, and because your entire musculoskeletal system is softening, injury may occur.

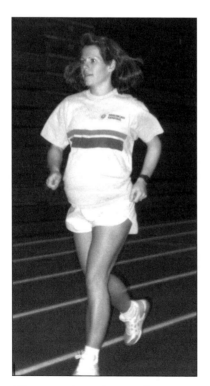

It happened to me. I developed a tendonitis of the ankle region at about sixteen weeks into my pregnancy. At the time, I was surprised at the sudden onset of the injury, but now I realize that it was probably due to a combination of factors: connective tissue changes, change in my running gait, and the additional few pounds of weight. I was able to cycle and swim for a few weeks and then started Stairmaster® workouts. I returned to running when all pain was gone and bought a new pair of running shoes that were softer and provided more support.

Proper warm up and stretching is essential to any workout in pregnancy (See Chapter 5). You need to listen to early warning signs, especially pain during or after a workout. This is not the time to run through or ignore a body signal.

Your running gait may change as your pregnancy advances.

Third Trimester

▶ *Varicosities*

The development of varicosities in the leg or vulvar area during pregnancy is more apt to occur if there is a family history or genetic predisposition. Rapid weight gain or tight restrictive clothing contributes to the problem. Also, progesterone, one of pregnancy's hormones, plays a role by causing the relaxation of the vein walls and the surrounding smooth muscles. Further pressure is placed on the pelvic veins by the expanded blood volume and the weight of the growing uterus.

If you have been physically active prior to pregnancy, you may be less apt to develop varicose veins. During pregnancy, exercise such as running and aerobics will help to improve circulation in the pelvic region and legs. If painful varicosities should develop, consider shortening an exercise routine or changing to another form of activity (less weight bearing).

You can obtain some relief by elevating your legs periodically during the day or by wearing supportive hose. You can provide support to the vulvar varices by wearing two snugly placed sanitary pads with a sanitary belt.

▶ *Swelling*

Most women will develop some mild swelling of the ankles or feet at some time during the pregnancy. Your growing uterus puts pressure on the blood vessels which return fluid from the legs. Restrictive clothing around the ankles, legs, or pelvic area impedes circulation and prolonged standing causes swelling in your legs and ankles. Swelling is usually most noticeable at the end of the day or in warm weather.

Adequate hydration (eight to ten glasses of liquid a day) helps the kidneys to work more effectively and reduces swelling. You can help by elevating your legs periodically, by avoiding crossing your legs, and by wearing comfortable supportive shoes, especially when exercising. I found that in the last few weeks of pregnancy, I was more comfortable running in a shoe with flexible uppers and more cushioning in the sole.

▶ *Braxton Hicks Contractions*

Braxton Hicks contractions usually begin sometime after the twentieth week of pregnancy. They are a painless tightening of the muscles in the uterus and become more frequent in the last month. Braxton Hicks differ from labor contractions because they are sporadic and non-rhythmic. Sometimes it is difficult to distinguish between Braxton Hicks contractions and premature labor or labor. If they occur more than four in an hour or with any kind of pain, you should notify your health care provider.

You can think of Braxton Hicks contractions as a "warm-up" session for labor. Changing your position or activity may stop the tightening of the uterine muscles. If they occur during exercise, stop or slow down and concentrate on slow deep breathing. This is an opportunity to listen to the signals your body is sending and "tune in." Runners may experience these tightenings while running. Slowing down or walking for a few minutes should help.

A Note To Fathers

Fathers-to-be play a significant role in a woman's feelings about herself in pregnancy. As a "partner in reproduction," you also need to learn as much as you can about the physical as well as emotional changes of pregnancy. Patience and understanding are the key words during the next nine months. Listen to your partner's concerns and appreciate the tremendous responsibility she is assuming in nurturing the baby's growth. As the most significant person in her life, you need to offer words of encouragement and support. I can remember asking my husband if I looked "big" in my eighth month. (I was feeling huge and didn't think I could possibly get any bigger.) His response was, "You look great!" At those critical moments when her self-esteem is teetering, she will need some ego boosting.

Fathers-to-be are also going through a change in identity. You are essentially on the outside of the construction site, but your concerns may be very similar. You will find yourself concerned about the health of the developing fetus and your partner, apprehensive about labor and delivery as well as the impact of parenthood and lifestyle changes. Talking about all these concerns will help you both get through the next nine months. Partners can even adopt a "pregnant status." Why not strive for a healthier diet, avoid alcohol, and spend time exercising together? A teamwork approach can start now and blossom during parenthood.

Your Changing Body — Your Changing Self

As you can see, your body will be changing tremendously during the next nine months. Carrying a child and giving birth is probably one of the most powerful experiences we will have in our lives. It is a period of both tremendous physical and emotional transformation — as we begin to integrate ourselves into the upcoming role of caretaker and parent. Our sense of self begins to change as our bodies change. There are new sensations, limitations, and opportunities for self-awareness. Part of this emotional adjustment is body image. Our once familiar "self" suddenly encounters the "pregnant self," and for some women these images can create a conflict.

► *Body Image*

Our society places heavy emphasis on the "ideal" female body — the firm, trim figure — and this ideal frequently compels many women to exercise. Some of you have worked hard through diet and exercise to get to this ideal state, or at least close to it. Now you are pregnant, and even if anticipated and met with joy, your pregnancy brings on the body changes we just discussed, and such changes may be at odds with your vision.

It is easy to think that you will maintain control with diet and more exercise — the same way you did before you were pregnant. You hope that continued exercise will be your salvation to restore you to your slim state after nine months of expansion. Many women fear getting bigger and then staying that way after the baby.

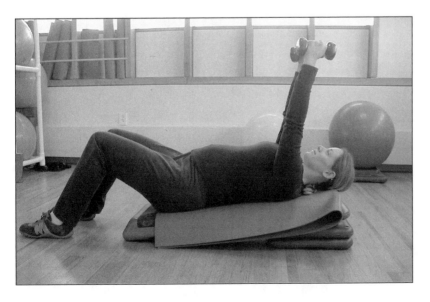

Exercise can build self-confidence as your body changes.

Our culture offers limited support on this topic. The "ideal" female image is in direct contrast to the basic biology of being female. If you allow yourself to accept this image, pregnancy may become a frustrating barrier to staying trim, fit, and athletic.

► *Bridging The Gap*

I encourage women to learn as much as possible about their growing, changing bodies. This knowledge will help you gain a sense of trust in your body as it adapts to pregnancy. The web is loaded with pregancy information. Libraries and bookstores are brimming with books on the topic. Share this information with your partner. Talk about all your sensations and changes. Talk with other women, especially other pregnant women and new mothers. Attend childbirth preparation classes with your partner for the opportunity to learn more about your pregnancy and to be around other couples like yourselves. Staying physically active and enjoying the benefits of exercise will help you bridge the gap and enjoy cooperating with your body for the next nine months.

What Others Say

Here are some comments from women like yourselves who exercised during their pregnancies:

"Exercise allowed me to deal with my changing body more easily. I felt like I could control one aspect of my life."

"I felt stronger and more confident about my pregnancy because of exercise."

"Exercise helped my physical and emotional upkeep."

"It (exercise) gave me emotional strength in dealing with the hormonal mood swings."

"I felt a little more in control of my body which seemed so out of my control."

"Exercise really lifted my spirits and helped me feel positive about getting larger."

"I felt strong. I had more stamina and endurance and a positive attitude."

Here are some comments from their partners:

"Don't discourage your wife from exercising ... they need it for their mental well-being."

"Encourage exercise but also make sure they (pregnant women) cooperate with what their bodies are telling them."

"I encouraged her to do whatever made her feel good."

"I was happy that my wife continued her exercise program because I could see the benefits she gained from it, but I was concerned that she not overdue it."

► *Emotional Passage*

The early signs of pregnancy, the breast tenderness, nausea, or fatigue, signal the mysterious beginnings of new life. What follows are more changes. Some are not so subtle. Vigorous kicking or lower backache can be the ever-constant reminders of your connection to the growing fetus inside. It is inevitable that conflicts will develop between your needs (e.g., sleep, back relief) and the needs of the fetus.

Exercise and body awareness can help calm the conflicts and nurture this connection. Women who engage in regular exercise are well attuned to their body and the signals that it sends. Physical activity or athletic competition provides us an opportunity to listen to the signals our body might be sending that warn about overtraining or pain, or about possible injury. This increased body awareness may help you better cope with the variety of physiological changes that you will encounter in your pregnancy.

The exercise goals of pregnancy are to maintain a safe level of fitness for you and your unborn baby. With these goals, an exercise program can help improve your body image and provide a sense of well-being and self confidence as your body changes.

"I felt great during all three of my pregnancies. I never had any morning sickness, back pain or any of the usual complaints. I did suffer from varicose veins but the doctor told me that running was probably the best thing for the circulation of my veins."
Runner and mother of three

Chapter 3

Safety First - Exercise Guidelines

*I*f you exercise regularly, you have likely discovered the physical, psychological as well as social benefits of physical activity. There are different rewards for each of us. We're out there running, cycling, or swimming to maintain cardiovascular fitness, to strengthen our bones and muscles, to control weight, and to seek mental relaxation. We like the "mental high" we feel after an invigorating run or aerobics class — the release of endorphins, the hormones which help to control pain and elevate our moods. Besides this sense of well being, we've found that staying fit can be a lot of fun. Lasting friendships are formed while circling the track, cycling around the countryside, or turning laps in a pool. Many active couples share the same love and enthusiasm for a particular sport or activity.

With the news of your pregnancy, all these "payoffs" of exercise that you have been enjoying need not cease. Yet, it is common for both you and your partner to wonder, "What exercise is safe for the next nine months?" When I first learned of my pregnancy, I was both thrilled and concerned — I wanted to know everything about my pregnancy, and, like other physically active women, I was eager to know how exercise might fit into the journey ahead. Let me share some of the things I learned.

How Exercise May Benefit Women And Babies *

- Increased circulation
- Avoidance of excessive weight gain
- Decreased fatigue
- Improved posture
- Decreased risk of blood clots, varicose veins, leg cramping, and swelling
- Decreased nausea
- Less low back pain
- Reduced risk of gestational diabetes
- Reduced risk of preeclampsia
- Shortened labor
- Increased comfort in third trimester
- Enhanced postpartum recovery
- Diminished depression

* Each woman's pregnancy experience is unique. While some realize many of these benefits, others do not.

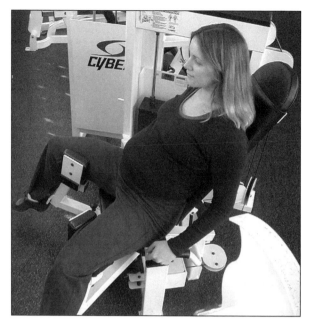

There is no evidence to suggest that you should stop exercising just because you are pregnant.

While there have been a lot of studies addressing exercise and pregnancy, most of the early work was done with pregnant animals, raising questions about just how valid the findings were for pregnant women. Most of the initial concerns have been put to rest. There is no reason to stop exercising just because you are pregnant.

So, pregnancy is not an excuse to "gestate" and become a couch potato, but neither is it a time to start up a strenuous sport or train for the Olympics. As we shall see, the majority of you can continue to do most types of activities, adjusting to your body's changes over the next nine months. It is important to honestly assess your own level of fitness and design an exercise plan with the guidance of your health care provider.

Suggestions for Exercise in Pregnancy
- All women should be encouraged to participate in aerobic and strength-conditioning exercise as part of a healthy lifestyle during their pregnancy
- Reasonable goals of aerobic conditioning in pregnancy should be to maintain a good fitness level throughout pregnancy without trying to reach peak fitness level or train for athletic competition
- Women should choose activities that will minimize the risk of loss of balance and fetal trauma
- Women should be advised that adverse pregnancy or neonatal outcomes are not increased for exercising women
- Initiation of pelvic floor exercises in the immediate postpartum period may reduce the risk of future urinary incontinence
- Women should be advised that moderate exercise during lactation does not affect the quantity or composition of breast milk or impact on fetal growth.

Royal College of Obstetricians and Gynaecologists (RCOG) January 2006

Exercise And Pregnancy Guidelines

Until 1985, there were no written guidelines for exercise in pregnancy. The American College of Obstetricians and Gynecologists (ACOG) published a bulletin in May of 1985, entitled "Exercise During Pregnancy and the Postnatal Period." This educational bulletin addressed a broad section of the population and was to be used as a guide for health care providers.

These early guidelines had some strict limitations. The bulletin advised women to keep their heart rate at 140 beats per minute and not engage in strenuous exercise for more than fifteen minutes. Adhering to those parameters, a well-conditioned woman would hardly be breaking into sweat. Health care providers relied heavily on this bulletin and given the medical-legal atmosphere, were reluctant to deviate from the prescribed recommendations, even for very fit women.

In 1994, ACOG altered the guidelines to move away from target heart rate and instead, use perceived exertion (See RPE later in this chapter) as a guide. In January 2002, ACOG issued new guidelines which continue to support exercise.

"Recreational and competitive athletes with uncomplicated pregnancies can stay active during pregnancy while modifying their usual exercise routines as medically indicated."   American College of Obstetricians and Gynecologists — 2002

The American College of Sports Medicine (ACSM) has also voiced their opinion on exercise and pregnancy, issuing recommendations in 2000 which are very supportive of exercise during pregnancy. The ACSM emphasizes the importance of developing an exercise program in consultation with your health care provider.

"...(P)articipation in regular weight-bearing exercise has been shown to improve maternal fitness, restrict weight gain without compromising fetal growth, and hasten postpartum recovery. In addition, the psychological benefits of exercise are undeniable, and should be nurtured by all who care for pregnant women." American College of Sports Medicine — 2000

These guidelines allow for a more individualized approach to exercise and encourage health care providers to help a woman develop an exercise program based on her current level of fitness and the health of her pregnancy. While they serve as a great general resource for pre-natal exercise, some experts believe the guidelines are too conservative. It is therefore best to talk with your health care provider about your exercise regime and to listen carefully to your body. Let's take a look at how your body adapts to exercise during pregnancy and some of the areas of concern for you and your baby.

Body Changes And Exercise

Pregnancy, as you learned in the last chapter, causes tremendous changes in your body. Your blood volume, cardiac output (amount of blood your heart pumps with each beat), and resting pulse all increase to help support the growing needs of the fetus as well as your own increase in size. This is all happening while you are resting and not even exercising. What happens when you start to run or cross country ski?

When you exercise, you will become aware of some of the changes occurring in your heart and lungs due to pregnancy. You most likely will feel breathless or short of breath as you begin to exercise because the uterus displaces the diaphragm upwards allowing for a smaller volume of air to fill the lungs. In addition, your brain signals the need to breathe faster since your carbon dioxide level will be higher because you are also eliminating CO_2 for the fetus.

Despite this shortness of breath, your body can adapt to moderate levels of exercise, especially if you are physically fit before becoming pregnant. As you might expect, your exercise performance will decline as your pregnancy advances. This seems to be more noticeable in weight bearing activities such as running versus a non-weight bearing exercise like cycling or swimming. All of the women I spoke with noticed this, especially in the last trimester of their pregnancies.

Change Your Workout Focus
"My cardio suffers in the first stages of my pregnancies and catching my breath is difficult, so I had to listen to my body and slow down. When riding indoors, I became overheated really easily, so I kept a fan in front of me and drank twice as much water. My workout focus changed from one of achievement and improvement to one of maintenance. I worked at a lower heart rate and began to use the perceived rate of exertion scale to monitor my exercise." Leah, Spinning® instructor and mother of two.

The cardiovascular changes in pregnancy are not only influenced by the duration, intensity, and type of exercise you are performing, but also by the position of your body. For example, you may, late in your pregnancy, feel faint or dizzy when lying on your back. This is called supine hypotension and is caused

Train For Your Pregnancy
A world-class runner didn't think of herself as an "athlete" while pregnant. Instead she looked at her pregnancy as though she were "in training" for a pregnancy and delivery of a healthy baby. She cut back her running from 70 miles a week to 4 to 5 easy miles a day. In the final weeks she reduced this to 1.5 to 2 miles a day. Sometimes she rode her bike while her husband, an Olympic marathoner, ran. She delivered a six and a half pound healthy baby girl.

by the enlarged uterus putting pressure on the vena cava, a main vein through which blood flows from the body back to the heart. The condition is more prevalent in larger women carrying big babies. If you are exercising, say doing crunches, you are highly unlikely to have supine hypotension. You can immediately relieve the symptoms by shifting on to your side. Prolonged standing without moving can cause similar problems due to a pooling of blood in your legs. As we note in Chapter 8, there are many ways to change exercises later in pregnancy to avoid any possible hypotension issues.

One of the most obvious changes in pregnancy is a steady shift in your center of gravity. Fortunately these changes occur gradually over time and we are "adapting" daily. Nevertheless, it is probably best to avoid activities where loss of balance may be dangerous. It's just good sense, even if you are adept, to avoid such things as riding technical mountain bike trails, tackling difficult downhill ski runs, or taking your horse over jumps. As you'll see throughout this book, there are many safe exercise alternatives for pregnant women.

Faye, a mother of two, is a swing dancer who continued to dance at a high level throughout each pregnancy.

> *"I think being fit made me feel better about the way I looked and the way I moved. As a dancer, I had become increasingly aware of how I move, and this helped as my body became bigger. I also had very strong abdominal muscles, and I think that helped me avoid back problems, which were never an issue in either pregnancy. Being active definitely helped with weight control. I also think that partner dancing as a form of exercise during pregnancy has an added advantage of being an activity that the parents can do together."*

A less obvious change is the relaxation of your joints and ligaments due to pregnancy hormones. This looseness of ligaments makes you more vulnerable to strains or sprains during exercise. This is especially true for weight bearing activities such as running or aerobics. Lower back pain, relatively common in pregnancy, is partly due to a relaxation of your lower back ligaments. (As noted earlier, women who exercise have less low back pain.) You can compensate for these changes by modifying your exercise patterns such as avoiding exercises like double leg raises and straight-leg toe touches that increase the bend in your back. (Prior to pregnancy, you will want to aim for overall body strength and conditioning. Concentrate on your abdominal and back muscles. Practice good posture and proper lifting and bending techniques. The payoff will be a more comfortable pregnancy with less risk of injury.)

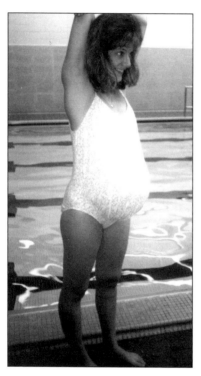

You "adapt" daily to the steady shift in your center of gravity.

Because of all the chemical changes taking place to meet the demands of pregnancy, your basal metabolic rate with normally be higher than before you were pregnant. This will cause you to feel warmer. Then, when you exercise, you will feel even warmer. How does your body get rid of this heat when you exercise in pregnancy? You sweat. Your increased blood volume helps to cool you and the fetus by transporting warmed blood towards your skin's surface where it is cooled. Sweating makes you feel cooler as water evaporates on your skin's surface. Since your body surface increases in pregnancy (added weight), this cooling response is enhanced even more. Women who are physically fit seem better able to stay cooler during exercise. A fit woman's cardiovascular system does a better job of moving blood to working muscles and to the skin's surface for cooling. Trained athletes sweat sooner and sweat more, thus staying cooler than untrained exercisers. But, regardless of your fitness, this is no license to ignore the risk of overheating, especially during early pregnancy.

What is the chance of overheating during exercise and how might this effect the fetus? Vigorous exercise for long periods of time can raise your core body temperature, which in turn causes the temperature of the fetus to rise. The critical temperature is in excess of 100.4 degrees F (38 degrees C). As noted earlier, take steps to avoid overheating to decrease the risks of problems. Limit your outdoor activity in very hot or humid conditions or head for the pool or an air-conditioned health club. Drink plenty of water to avoid dehydration. Avoid hot tubs, saunas and whirlpools, especially in early pregnancy. Don't exercise if you have an illness with a fever. Play it safe.

When you exercise, you need to eat enough to meet the basic metabolic needs of pregnancy plus the energy requirements of your physical activity. In general, you should eat to appetite and eat a well-balanced diet. Adequate weight gain

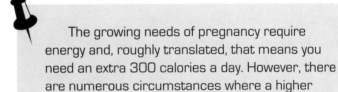

The growing needs of pregnancy require energy and, roughly translated, that means you need an extra 300 calories a day. However, there are numerous circumstances where a higher caloric intake becomes necessary, for instance:
- <19 years of age
- excessive vomiting in the first trimester
- close pregnancy spacing
- failure to gain 20 lbs by the 20th week.

Whenever additional calories are needed protein intake must also increase.

is a good gauge or indicator that you are keeping up with your caloric needs. Complex carbohydrates are an excellent source of energy and best replace the nutrients lost during exercise. (See Chapter 4)

What About The Fetus?

Prior to pregnancy, your exercise goals and mood dictated your physical activity. Now that you are pregnant, you need to consider the passenger on board. The health and well being of the fetus is the focus of numerous studies in pregnancy. Let's see how your exercise affects the fetus.

► *Blood Flow and Oxygen Supply*

During exercise, there is a shift of blood flow from your internal organs (including the uterus) to your working muscles (arms, legs). Conflicting results in studies examining blood flow to the uterus prohibit us from drawing any definite conclusions. We do know that the diversion of blood flow from the uterus is probably lessened due to some of the physiological changes in a normal, healthy pregnancy. Your expanded blood volume, increased cardiac output (you pump more per beat), and relaxation of your blood vessels helps to compensate and maintain blood flow to the uterus during moderate levels of exercise. So for safety's sake, exercise at moderate levels — leave the vigorous, prolonged workouts until after pregnancy.

The fetal heart rate is a widely used method for studying the well being of the fetus. While some studies have shown lowered fetal heart rate (bradycardia) during exercise by unfit women, there is little evidence to show fetal heart rate anomalies with fit women. However, you should always avoid prolonged and intense workouts and clear any exercise program with your health care provider.

➤ *Birth Weight*

Studies comparing babies' birth weights in active and inactive women have been contradictory. As noted earlier, some studies have suggested that women who exercise at high intensities throughout pregnancy have smaller babies. Birth weight for the exercisers was about 300 grams lower, however, the babies were not stunted in their growth — they had less body fat. Dr. James Clapp has found that bigger babies occur when women exercise vigorously in the beginning of pregnancy and then cut down or stop toward the end. (The reason for this is that the active first half of pregnancy increases the size of the placenta which in turn feeds the fetus.) At best, we can conclude that exercise type (i.e., weight-bearing versus non-weight-bearing) and intensity may account for some of the discrepancy. In general, adequate maternal weight gain and appropriate fetal growth are good indicators that your exercise program falls into the "safe" category for the fetus.

Many active women want to know if exercise will cause a miscarriage, premature labor or developmental problems with the fetus. There is no evidence to suggest that moderate exercise in a healthy pregnancy will cause a miscarriage, alter development

Mary Anne ran during both her pregnancies. "I no longer ran for time. I would cut back immediately if I felt tired." She reduced her mileage each trimester and walked 3 to 4 miles a day the last six weeks because of what she described as shin discomfort. Though never diagnosed, it is likely that her anterolateral leg pain was due to swelling and distention of the fascia, the thin connective tissue, which covers the lower leg muscles. Walking was a wise alternative to running. After an hour and a half labor, Mary Anne had a healthy seven pound, six ounce boy.

of the fetus or put you at higher risk for premature labor. In fact, moderate activity in healthy, well-nourished, pregnant women can actually prevent some health problems like excessive weight gain, poor posture and lower back pain, fatigue and poor body image. Exercise also reduces risk for preeclampsia and gestational diabetes. (One study by Dempsey et al quotes a risk reduction of 50% in gestational diabetes and a 40% risk reduction for preeclampsia.) More research using large scale prospective studies is needed to better understand the effects of different types of exercise during pregnancy and the outcomes during labor and delivery as well as the effects of exercise during the postpartum period and lactation.

Sports And Activities To Avoid

Avoid any sport or activity which might cause trauma or serious injury to the abdomen. Even if you suffer only a mild injury to your abdomen, this could potentially have more serious consequences for the fetus such as abruption of the placenta (separation of the placenta from the wall of the uterus). Sports to avoid include hockey, soccer, hang gliding, boxing, fencing, water-skiing, and diving. Similarly, because of the risk of falling, I recommend that you stay away from downhill skiing, skate blading, rock climbing, and ice skating in the later months of pregnancy. (Being pregnant can make it difficult to treat injuries due to the potential risks to the fetus from drugs or anesthesia.) Scuba and deep sea diving can expose you to potentially dangerous pressure changes. In case of doubt, use your common sense.

What precautions should you take at high altitudes? The lack of oxygen at higher altitude can put additional stress on you and your fetus. Avoid altitudes over 10,000 feet during pregnancy. Don't hike or ski at elevations above 6,000 feet. Allow yourself three to four days to acclimate to the altitude prior to exercising.

Flying during pregnancy is safe but most airlines will not permit flying during your last month in case you go into labor naturally.

Workout Intensity Level

It is important to exercise at your fitness level. So how can you determine just what is your level of intensity? Target heart rate is a popular method to calculate exercise intensity but during pregnancy, your resting heart rate increases, so using target heart rate may not be the best way to measure your level of maximum intensity. A better measure of exercise intensity is the <u>Rating of Perceived Exertion</u> (RPE) as developed by Borg, a Swedish physiologist. Using this method, you can correlate your perceived activity level with exertion and aerobic activity. The scale goes from 6 to 20; 6 - 7 being very, very light workouts and 19 - 20 being very, very, hard. Try to be as close as possible to when estimating your feelings of exertion. During pregnancy, you should stay around 12-14, (somewhat hard) when exercising. At this intensity of exercise, you should be able to pass the "Talk Test" and easily carry on a conversation while exercising.

Rating Of Perceived Exertion Scale

How does the exercise feel?	Rating
	6
Very, very light	7
	8
Very light	9
	10
Fairly light	11
	12
Somewhat Hard	13
	14
Hard	15
	16
Very hard	17
	18
Very, very hard	19
	20

Warning Signs

After establishing your exercise program with the guidance of your health provider, you need to recognize warning signs that may alert you to a problem. The following signs and symptoms tell you to stop exercising and to consult your provider.

• Pain Unfortunately, many well-conditioned athletes are used to discomfort during workouts. You need to slow down and listen to your body as it moves from discomfort to pain. "No pain, no gain" does not apply during pregnancy.

• Bleeding Any vaginal bleeding or spotting at any time in pregnancy means STOP and contact your health care provider immediately.

- Dizziness, Shortness of Breath, Palpitations, Faintness, or very Rapid Heartbeat   Any one of these symptoms is a signal to stop exercising.
- Pubic Pain   This may signal irritation, or if persistent, a more serious injury to the pubic bone due to loosening of ligaments.
- Rupture of Uterine Membranes (Leaking Amniotic Fluid) or Regular Uterine Contractions*   Stop exercising. Call your health care provider.

* It is important for pregnant women to distinguish between normal "Braxton Hicks" or "pregnancy" contractions with those that might indicate preterm labor. Basically, any contractions that cause pain or significant discomfort just above the pubic bone need to be checked by a health care provider. Contractions that are painless and just feel "tight" are normal. If you have more than six of these each hour you can slow them down by lying on your left side and drinking twelve ounces of water. It is normal to have an increase in Braxton Hicks contractions after exercise, after sex, and also at the end of the day, especially if you have been on your feet a lot.

Use the "Talk Test" to monitor your workouts during pregnancy.

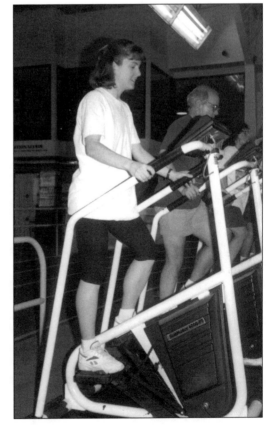

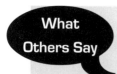

A former collegiate All-American cross country runner and mother of three tells about how she exercised through her pregnancies:

"I have done a lot of research regarding running and pregnancy but I think that really listening to my body and applying common sense were the best guides. I cut down on my mileage while pregnant. For example, before one of my pregnancies, I was running about 55 miles/week and I cut that down to 35-40. I ceased doing intervals and any running that would boost my heart rate too much or cause me to get dehydrated or overheated. On any given day, especially toward the end of the pregnancies, if I had too much cramping or too many Braxton Hicks contractions, I would walk. I had a lot of Braxton Hicks contractions when I ran and if they became too much on any given day, then I would fast walk, swim or call it a day. Toward the end of my pregnancies, my mileage would drop to maybe 20 miles per week. I had full support from my doctors for my exercise routines.

I had pretty easy pregnancies with no complications so they never told me to stop running.

I did a few races but I ran the same pace as I did in workouts (in other words, I jogged). I had no interest in pushing myself that hard while pregnant. I manually check my heart rate but as a general rule, if I can talk to my running friends while running, then I find I am not taxing my body too much.

I felt great during all three of my pregnancies. I never had any morning sickness, back pain or any of the usual complaints. I did suffer from varicose veins but the doctor told me that running was probably the best thing for the circulation of my veins.

I had three natural childbirths and I feel that many years of interval training readied me for the contractions, intense pain and the duration of labor."

A former competitive distance runner (three time member of US Junior National Team) and mother of four tells how she learned from each pregnancy:

"Before my first pregnancy, I was running about 40 miles per week but dropped that significantly when I found out I was pregnant and stopped running entirely by eight weeks. I walked and cross country skied through twenty-four weeks. Overall I had trouble adjusting to the feeling of being pregnant and what was safe to do while pregnant, and overall I would say I was a bit paranoid and insecure.

Being an athlete influenced my pregnancy experiences. It threw me for a loop the first time around because I was so used to being able to control my body. I needed to learn how to relax and trust my body rather than force it into submission. In subsequent pregnancies I feel I had much more trust in myself and was able to combine that trust with some of the more positive attributes of being a runner, such as unquestioning belief in my strength and endurance. I think this allowed me to break free of the insecurities I had in my first pregnancy so that I could actively seek the pregnancy and birth experience I really wanted".

Setting Your Own Guidelines

As you read this book, you'll hear from women who continued to run, cycle, canoe, or ski throughout their pregnancies. You'll hear from others who had to slow down, change activities, or even stop exercising altogether. Just as each of us is different, each of our pregnancies will be different. That's why you must individualize your exercise program and set it up under the guidance of your health provider. Here are some exercise tips to consider when you do:

1. Listen to your body. Now is the time to tune in to all the signals and cues.
2. Be prepared to adapt and modify your program. Be flexible!
3. Rest. Any exercise program should be balanced by adequate rest.
4. Eat! Maintain a balanced diet with adequate calories. Let your appetite guide you.
5. Avoid high intensity workouts. Slow and easy ... keep it 12-14 on the RPE scale.
6. Avoid overheating and drink plenty of fluids.
7. Recognize warning signs to stop exercising.

"*I was extremely nauseous well into the second trimester during both pregnancies. This only occasionally interfered with running, but I had to be very careful to stay hydrated. Physically I felt great.*"

Runner and mother of two

Chapter 4

Nutrition

Your pregnancy will be a period in your life when you will be showered with attention. You'll get congratulatory greetings, inquiries about your health, comments on how big or small you are, and keen observations on every morsel you put in your mouth. Discerning eyes will never fail to capture you when you are surrendering to that dish of ice cream or an extra slice of pizza. But it's up to you to "eat for two" wisely.

What you eat or don't eat during pregnancy is important: it affects your health and the growing needs of your developing baby. For example, a diet deficient in essential nutrients may result in a low birth weight baby who is at risk for delivery complications, infection, or impaired intelligence. Conversely, a well-balanced diet, both before and during pregnancy, increases your chances of delivering a healthy normal weight baby. No one's diet is perfect, but certainly during your pregnancy you should plan your diet carefully and focus on "quality."

Ideally, the time for you to establish a healthy pattern of eating is <u>before</u> pregnancy. There is evidence that a diet deficient in folic acid may contribute to neural tube defects (spina bifida). Current guidelines recommend that childbearing women should consume 0.4 mg of folic acid a day. You can meet this by eating a diet rich in leafy vegetables, whole grains, eggs, oranges and legumes, however, a daily multivitamin is recommended to ensure adequate intake of folic acid. It is best to begin taking the vitamin at least a month before becoming pregnant.

Your iron consumption is also important during pregnancy as it leads to healthy blood and strong bones and teeth. During pregnancy your iron level will be tested for anemia, a condition that causes fatigue. While proteins, dried fruits, legumes and nuts are good sources of iron, a prenatal vitamin will again help to maintain a consistent level of iron in your system.

Eating For Two

Most of you have probably eagerly planned for your pregnancy. At the same time, if you are physically active, you have concerns about how your pregnancy will affect your body. In particular, you are probably worried about weight gain and how you will lose the weight afterwards. Of the women I see in my practice, one of their biggest fears is getting "fat" and then not losing the weight because of lack of exercise due to the demands of parenting.

Are you concerned about weight gain? It's not unusual — many physically active and athletic women exercise to control their weight. Competitive athletes are keenly aware of weight gain and may restrict themselves calorically by following a very low fat diet. Because of this, these women may also be deficient in certain vitamins and minerals, especially iron, even before they conceive.

The apprehension of becoming fat probably exists for most of us during our lifetime, sometimes starting with adolescence and continuing into adulthood. During pregnancy, this concern can be magnified. I know that during my pregnancy I didn't want to gain excessive weight because I wanted to stay fit both during and after the pregnancy. On the other hand, my goal was to gain "nutritiously" and grow a healthy baby.

For the average woman, weight gain during pregnancy is usually between 25 and 35 pounds, but everyone is different. For example, some women gain more in the first trimester because they eat to control nausea. Others gain eight to ten pounds in four-week period between 24 and 28 weeks due to blood volume expansion. Occasionally women lose a few pounds in the last month despite eating normally. So your weight gain situation will be unique to you and will be something you review with your health care provider throughout your pregnancy.

Quality Counts

Eating a healthy diet during your pregnancy will reap many rewards for you and your baby. A balanced diet will help improve your mood swings and boost your energy level while it improves the odds of delivering a healthy baby.

This "healthy eating" responsibility may feel overwhelming at times, especially if you had an unbalanced diet before pregnancy. Why not think of pregnancy as training for an athletic event — the birth of your baby? Make a proper diet an integral part of your training.

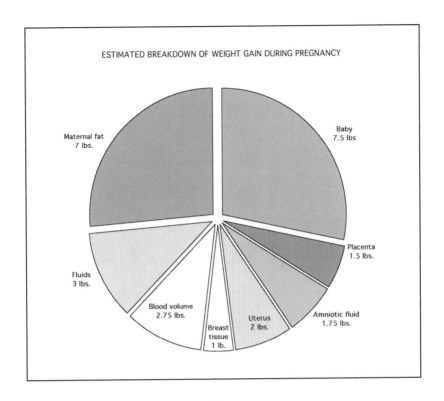

ESTIMATED BREAKDOWN OF WEIGHT GAIN DURING PREGNANCY

Maternal fat
7 lbs.

Baby
7.5 lbs

Placenta
1.5 lbs.

Fluids
3 lbs.

Blood volume
2.75 lbs.

Breast
tissue
1 lb.

Uterus
2 lbs.

Amniotic fluid
1.75 lbs.

Expectant Eating

In pregnancy, we require an additional 300 calories a day, for the growing fetus and for the energy needs of just being pregnant. When you think about it, 300 calories does not really add up to a feeding frenzy. A bran muffin and a cup of yogurt add up to this "extra." The challenge is to create a balanced energizing diet. The first step is to look at your current diet. Keep track of everything you eat or drink for several days (be honest!). You might want to review it against the new USDA MyPyramid food guidance system (www.mypyramid.gov) which provides a lot of options to help you make healthy food choices and stay active. Here are some of its recommendations:

Grains   Eat at least 3 ounces of whole-grain cereals, rice, or pasta every day. (1 ounce is about 1 slice of bread, about 1 cup of breakfast cereal, or 1/2 cup of cooked rice, cereal, or pasta)

Vegetables   Eat more dark-green veggies like broccoli, spinach, and other dark leafy greens. Eat more orange vegetables like carrots and sweet potatoes. Eat more dry beans and peas like pinto beans, kidney beans, and lentils.

Fruits   Eat a variety of fruit. Choose fresh, frozen, canned, or dried fruit. Go easy on fruit juices.

Milk   Go low fat or fat-free when you chose milk, yogurt, and other milk products. (If you don't or can't consume milk, chose lactose-free products or other calcium sources such as fortified foods and beverages.)

Meat & Beans   Choose low-fat or lean meats and poultry. Bake it, broil it, or grill it. Vary your protein routine – choose more fish, beans, peas, nuts, and seeds.

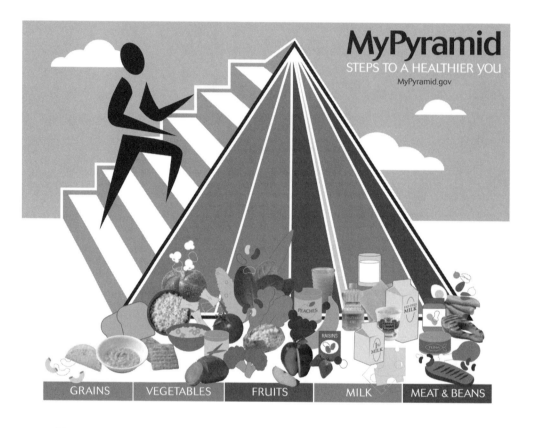

The new USDA MyPyramid food guidance system (www.mypyramid.gov) can help you make healthy food choices and stay active.

Diet For The Active Pregnancy

There has been little research on the nutritional needs of physically active women in pregnancy. The energy needs of active pregnant women vary with the type of activity you are performing, its duration, and your stage in the pregnancy. It is impossible to provide specific guidelines due to all of these variables. Basically, if you "eat to appetite" (eat when you are hungry, stop when you are full), you will fulfill the energy needs of your physical activity and growing needs of your baby. You should concentrate on complex carbohydrates (whole grain breads, cereals, rice, vegetables, dried beans and peas). Some pregnant women quit eating fish altogether due to concerns about mercury – but this may not be a healthy choice. Fish that is high in essential fatty acids promotes fetal brain development. (While there is controversy about mercury levels in tuna, you can find safe alternatives such as shrimp, salmon, clams, and tilapia.)

Foods To Avoid Or Limit During Pregnancy

Deli meats and unpasteurized cheeses should be avoided as they can contain listeria, a type of bacteria that is especially harmful to pregnant women and their unborn babies. Meats should not be eaten if they are not cooked or undercooked.

Many types of fish have a high mercury content that can be harmful to a baby's brain and nervous system. The highest levels of mercury are found in shark, swordfish, king mackerel and tilefish (also called golden or white snapper.) These types of fish should be avoided.

Tuna fish and canned tuna (especially white/albacore) should be limited to 2 servings or 12 oz a week. Fish with lower mercury levels are: shrimp, salmon, pollock, catfish and light tuna. Visit http://www.cfsan.fda.gov/~dms/admehg3.html to learn more about mercury in fish.

Salt intake, which is found in high amounts in processed foods such as soups, canned vegetables, chips and fast food, should be monitored as high sodium consumption can cause the body to retain water and therefore result in swelling, a problem that arises in the later stages of pregnancy.

Caffeine should be limited to a minimal amount such as a cup of coffee or a glass of soda. Large amounts of caffeine have been known to lead to low birth-weight babies. Caffeine also acts as a diuretic depleting your body of water.

Alcohol consumed by a pregnant woman goes into the blood stream and reaches the baby via its umbilical cord. Excessive consumption of alcohol can slow down the baby's growth, including brain development, and can result in birth defects. As it is not known exactly how much alcohol is harmful, it is recommended that pregnant women abstain from alcohol consumption during pregnancy.

U.S. Department of Health & Human Services. 2005. Pregnancy and a Healthy Diet. Washington, D.C.

Your weight gain will help you determine if you are taking in enough calories. If you begin to lose weight, or fail to gain, this is an indicator that you need to examine closely your diet and make the necessary changes to gain adequate weight. Reviewing a two or three day diet recall is an easy way to do this. If you are lactose intolerant or do not drink milk, you may need to take a calcium supplement. A discussion with your health provider about your exercise program and diet is important. You want to be sure that both you and your baby are gaining and "growing nutritiously."

After The Baby

One of the first concerns of most women after delivery is getting back to their prepregnancy weight. Remember, it took you nine months to gain the weight so it will take a bit of time to lose it. A common mistake some women make is to starve themselves to achieve a rapid weight loss. This approach has a price to pay.

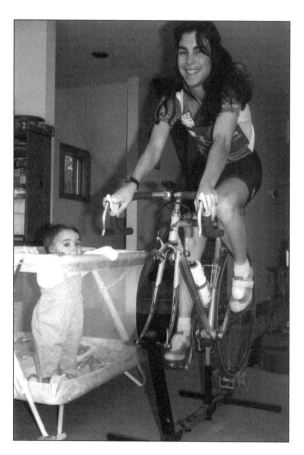

Exercise and nutrition A.B. (After Baby) takes some extra planning.

In the weeks following delivery, your body is undergoing some significant changes. Your uterus is shrinking, blood volume is decreasing, and hormones are changing to lactation hormones if you are breastfeeding or dropping to their nonpregnant levels if you are not. All of this change, plus the arrival of your new baby who depends on you and your partner for everything, can feel overwhelming. Some women experience "postpartum blues." These "down" feelings can occur as early as the third day postpartum or any time during the first year. Two of the major causes are the tremendous shift in hormones and fatigue. Interrupted sleep is one of the biggest challenges new parents have to cope with. We'll talk more about this later, but a healthy diet will help you survive these first few months.

If you are breastfeeding, you need an additional 400-500 calories a day. This extra energy will assure an adequate milk supply. Breastfeeding demands the same scrutiny of your diet you had during pregnancy. You can excrete substances from what you eat or drink in your breast milk. Limiting your caffeine or alcohol intake is wise. Be sure to question the safety of over the counter or prescription drugs with your health provider. It is advisable to take continue taking a prenatal vitamin while nursing.

Be sure to talk to your health care provider about both your exercise program and your diet. It's not always easy to be objective about your own eating habits, especially when that hot fudge sundae is screaming your name, so it's good to get an outside opinion. Your nutrition game plan is an important part of a fit pregnancy.

"I kept my peace of mind and was more concerned with the baby's and my health than staying in tip-top condition." Rower and mother of two

Chapter 5

Stretching

As a fit woman, you are well aware of the importance of proper warm-up, stretching and cool down routines in your exercise program. Unfortunately, this awareness does not always get translated into practice. I know the excuses because I've used most of them: "I'm in a hurry — I'll stretch later — This feels too easy — I'd rather be working out." Now, during pregnancy, it's more important than ever to include a few simple routines into pregnancy and post-pregnancy fitness programs. Why risk injury by launching too quickly into a workout? Warming up and cooling down routines are a good investment of your time.

Warm-up/Cooldown Routines

In Chapter 2, we first mentioned that pregnancy hormones make your joints and ligaments more relaxed and vulnerable to injury. (You'll hear it again — it is important to keep in mind.) When you warm up, you raise the temperature of your muscles, route more blood to your muscles, and increase the synovial fluid (a fluid that lubricates) in your joints. You prepare your tendons, ligaments, and muscles for the work ahead.

Is stretching the same as warming up? No, it is not. After a brief warm-up, you can gently stretch the major muscles that you will be using in your workout. For instance, in running you would focus on your calf, quadriceps, and hamstring muscles before the run, saving the bulk of your stretching for after your workout when your muscles will be warmed and more flexible.

A warm-up can be as simple as jogging 5 to 10 minutes prior to running, doing a few easy laps in the pool, or spinning your wheels on the bike for a few miles. The idea is to slowly get specific muscles warmed up and ready for the workout.

Cooling down, or slowing down, is the best way to end your workout. Cooling down slowly lowers your heart rate and reduces muscle soreness. A slow jog around the corner, a few easy laps of breaststroke, or walking in place after aerobics is all it takes to lead into your post-exercise stretching routine. Towel off or change into dry clothes beforehand if necessary. Grab something to drink and start your stretching routine.

Proper Stretching

Like warm-ups and cooldowns, stretching is easy to skip over when you are short on time. However, now, more than ever, you should pledge to take the time to stretch. Stretching has a lot of positive benefits: it relaxes your muscles, promotes better circulation, and helps you stay flexible. It also keeps you focused on your changing body as you take the time to stretch specific muscle groups. Stretching relaxes your muscles and your mind.

Stretching is easy, but learn to do it properly. Improper stretching can cause injury to joints, ligaments or muscles during and after your pregnancy. Bob Anderson, in his book, *Stretching*, offers the following tips. Never force a stretch to the point of pain.

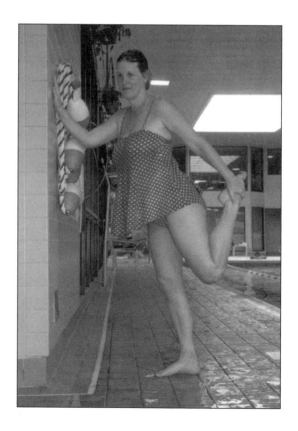

Stretching relaxes your muscles, promotes better circulation, and helps you stay flexible.

Avoid bouncing. Instead, try for a relaxed, slow stretch. Breathe in and out slowly and don't hold your breath. Begin a stretch by holding it for 10 to 30 seconds, then stretch a little further. You should feel some mild tension but not pain. Hold the stretch for another 10 to 30 seconds. Listen to your body along the way and make adjustments as necessary.

Pregnancy Stretches

There are some excellent books on stretching. A particularly good one is the forementioned *Stretching* by Bob Anderson (See Resource Section). Most likely you have your own stretching routine already in place that you can modify both during and after your pregnancy. The following are some stretches that are especially good during pregnancy.

► *Neck Rolls*
- Can be done sitting or standing
- Drop your head to the right, slowly roll your head forward and then to your left shoulder.
- Repeat several times.

► *Shoulder Rolls*
- Can be done sitting or standing.
- Move your right shoulder forward, upward and then down and back, making a full circle.
- Repeat with your left shoulder.
- Do 5 reps each side.

► *Arm Reaches*
- Stand or sit.
- Inhale as you raise your right arm above your head, stretching from the waist.
- Exhale as you bring your arm down.
- Repeat on the left side.
- Do 5 reps on each side.

► *Arm Stretches*

- Can be done standing or sitting.
- Raise your right arm over your head, bending it at the elbow, and place your hand on your back.
- Grab your elbow with your left hand and gently pull back.
- You should feel the stretch along your upper arm.
- Hold the stretch for 10 to 30 seconds, then stretch a little further for another 10 to 30 seconds.
- Repeat on your left arm.
- For the outer arm muscles, bring your right arm straight across your chest.
- Place your left hand on your elbow and gently pull your arm closer to your chest.
- Hold for 10 to 30 seconds and then stretch a little further for another 10 to 30 seconds.
- Repeat on your left arm.

► *Chest Stretch*

- Stand with your feet slightly apart.
- Lace your fingers together behind your back.
- Slowly lift your hands up behind you, pulling your shoulder blades together and keeping your head level.
- Hold for 10 to 30 seconds and then stretch a little further or another 10 to 30 seconds.

► *Pelvic Tilt-Standing*

- Stand comfortably.
- Inhale and relax. Exhale and pull your buttocks under and forward. Hold for the count of 5. You can also do this pressing the small of your back against a wall.
- Do 5 reps.

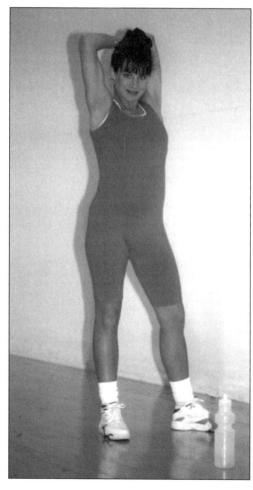

Arm stretches can be done standing or sitting.

► *Pelvic Tilt-Kneeling*

- Kneel on your hands and knees on a padded surface, making sure that your back is straight and parallel to the floor.
- Inhale and relax.
- Then, as you exhale, tuck your chin, pull your buttocks under and forward while feeling your abdomen tightening. Hold for the count of 5.
- Inhale as you lengthen your spine by returning your tailbone to the original position.
- Do 5 reps.

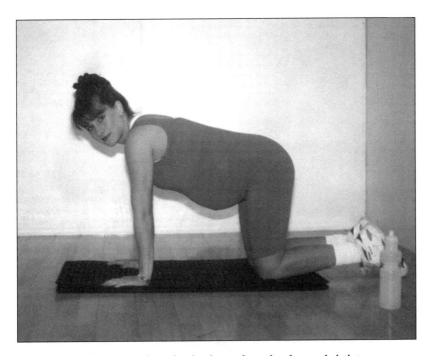

The pelvic tilt helps relieve backache and can be done while lying on your back, standing, or on your hands and knees.

► *Kegel Exercise*

- Helps to strengthen muscles that support your bladder, uterus, and rectum.
- Can be done lying down, sitting, or standing.
- Tighten and release the muscles around your vagina. (Try this exercise while urinating by starting and then stopping the flow of urine.)
- Work up to 25 contractions.

► *Wall Squats*

- Stand with your back, head, and shoulders against the wall.
- Pressing your lower back to the wall, squat as if you were going to sit down.
- Come up slowly, keeping your back and buttocks in contact with the wall.

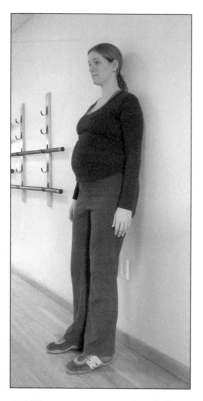 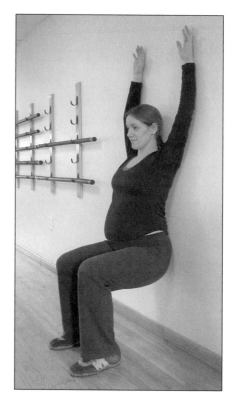

Wall squats are great for abdominal muscles, buttock muscles and thigh muscles. Note that the feet are 1-2 feet from the wall.

► *Butterfly/Groin Stretch*

- Sit on the floor with the soles of your feet together.
- Hold your ankles.
- Bring your feet as close to your body as comfortable while keeping your back straight.
- Inhale and relax. Exhale and lower yourself forward.

Hold the stretch easy for 10 to 30 seconds, then stretch a little further for another 10 to 30 seconds.

- Squatting is a good stretch for your inner thigh and calf muscles.
- Squat down, keeping your back straight.
- Keep your heels on the floor while you balance yourself evenly on flat feet.

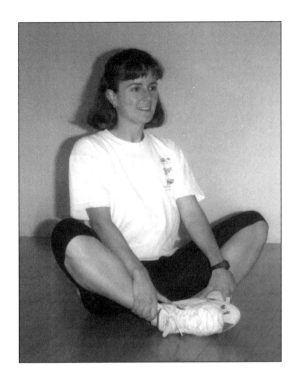

When doing the butterfly stretch you should feel a stretch in your inner thighs.

► *Leg Stretches*

- Sit on the floor with your left leg stretched out to the side, your foot flexed, and your other leg drawn in.
- Face forward and lean your body toward the outstretched leg.
- Lift your right arm over your head and with your left hand grasp your ankle or calf.
- Hold the stretch for 10 to 30 seconds, then stretch a little further for another 10 to 30 seconds, then repeat on the right side.

► *Side Leg Stretches*

- Lie on your right side with legs straight or with the lower leg bent at the knee.
- Support your head with your right hand and place your left hand in front of you.
- Inhale and relax.
- Keep your foot flexed as you raise your left leg as high as you can, then exhale as you slowly lower it.
- Repeat ten times then roll to your left side and repeat ten times.
- You can also do this with your top leg bent at the knee so your leg is at a right angle to your body. Keep your foot flexed as you raise and lower your leg.

➤ *Calf Stretches*

- Stand facing a wall.
- Bend one knee and bring it toward the wall.
- Keep your back leg straight with your foot facing forward.
- Press your heel to the floor.
- Feel the stretch in your calf muscle.
- Hold for 10 to 30 seconds then stretch a little further for another 10 to 30 seconds. Stretch the other calf.

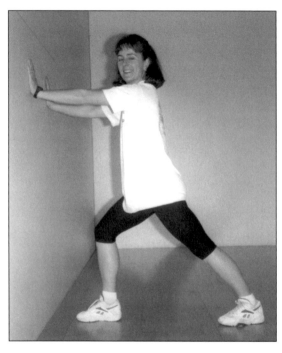

You can stretch your calf muscles against a wall or on a stair step.

➤ *Lunge Stretch*

- Bring your right leg forward and bend your knee, keeping your foot facing straight.
- Your leg should be at a right angle to the floor.
- Support your body with your hands on the floor.
- Stretch your left leg behind you while pushing your hips down toward the floor.
- Hold this stretch for 10 to 30 seconds.
- Switch legs and repeat.

Massage is a comforting technique which relieves muscle tension, improves flexibility and increases circulation. Many athletes include sport massage in their training as a way to promote recovery and reduce the risk of injury. Massage therapy helps remove lactic acid, a byproduct of anaerobic exercise, which is believed to cause muscle soreness. When done correctly, massage provides a feeling of relaxation and well being. A massage by your partner or friend offers relief to tense shoulders, lower backache and other pregnancy trouble spots. You can give yourself a "mini-massage" or treat yourself to a professional massage. Massage should be avoided if you have a history of phlebitis or blood clots.

➤ *Hamstrings*

- From a standing position, place your right foot in front of you.
- Push your heel into the floor as you pull your toes up toward you.
- Try to keep your leg straight and back flat. Bend your left leg for support.
- Feel the stretch along the back of your leg.
- Hold for 10 to 30 seconds, then stretch a little further to 10 to 30 seconds.
- Repeat with your right leg.

➤ *Quadriceps Stretch*

- Stand next to a wall or chair for support.
- Bend your left knee and with your right hand, pull your heel straight back toward your buttocks.
- Keep your thigh parallel to your other leg.
- Hold for 10 to 30 seconds and then stretch a little further for another 10 to 30 seconds.
- Repeat on your right leg.

Stretching feels good. Proper stretching relaxes your muscles, reduces tension, promotes circulation, keeps you flexible and prevents injury. Tailor your stretching routine to your own body signals and tight spots. For instance, as a runner you might focus more on your legs and hips. Swimmers and paddlers will want to stretch more of their upper bodies. No two bodies are the same and pregnancy will likely cause new "trouble spots," like your back, hips and pelvis. Easy stretching will offer relief and help you relax mentally and physically. It's time well spent.

"Almost every night, especially in the last trimester, I had to do some poses to stretch my hips and back so I would be able to sleep." Mother of two

Chapter 6

Pilates, Yoga, Exercise Ball

*E*xercises that focus on both the mind and body are great alternatives or additions to more physical, cardiovascular forms of exercise. While there are a host of such exercises out there, this chapter will focus on Pilates, yoga, and the exercise ball. Given that all these forms of exercise rely on relaxation, breathing, and strengthening of muscle groups, you will find that the disciplines use some of the same exercises.

Pilates

Pilates, a buzzword among gyms and sports clubs, is a mind-body form of exercise that can be tailored to pregnancy. Joseph Pilates created the form of exercise in the early 1900s as a means of body sculpting without the use of weights. The exercises focus on strengthening the abdominal muscles, pelvic area and buttocks, and back – areas that play an important role in pregnancy and labor and delivery.

> *"Everything should be smooth, like a cat. The exercises are done lying, sitting, kneeling, etc. to avoid excessive strain on the heart and lungs."* Joseph Pilates

Pilates is like yoga in its purposeful movement, but the exercises focus more on rhythmical movement than on holding a position. The movement is slow to allow for concentration, conscious breathing, and relaxation. While Pilates is a gentle form of exercise, some movements should be avoided or adapted during pregnancy. Look for classes and/or videos or books that are directed toward pregnancy; this is especially important for beginners. Below are some general guidelines for Pilates for the expectant mother, however, as each person's pregnancy is unique in discomfort and complications, you should consult an instructor or health provider regarding an appropriate regimen.

- Avoid movements that put too much on stress on abdominal and back muscles, areas that become more sensitive in later pregnancy.
- Avoid lying on your back (supine position) in the second and third trimesters as the position can cut off the oxygen supply to your baby.
- Breath awareness is at the heart of Pilates and you exhale with the movement to encourage relaxation. You should not be holding your breath at any time as it may lead to dizziness and/or nausea.
- Exercise at your comfort level recognizing that pregnancy causes a shift in balance and a loosening of ligaments.

Some Pilates Exercises

Exercises should be done on a mat. Three to five repetitions are recommended.

► *The Cat – Being on your hands and knees is a comfortable position during pregnancy taking the weight of the baby off of your back. This position also encourages your baby to drop into the desired head down position later in pregnancy.*

- Get on your hands and knees with a flat back like a tabletop. Your knees should be shoulder-width apart and in alignment with your hips.
- Breathe in, then breathe out while drawing on your abdominals to arch your back.
- Keep your head relaxed so that it falls between your straightened arms.
- Breathe in and return to the previous position with a flat back.
- Breathe out and arch your back so that it is concave dipping below your head and bottom.
- Breathe in and return to position.

The cat exercise, which stretches the entire back, is common to both Pilates and yoga.

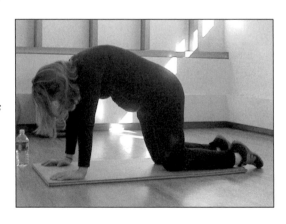

➤ *Back Strength – another position on hands on knees.*
- Lift and straighten one leg and the opposite arm (forming a half-X) and keep both limbs in line with your torso.
- Switch sides paying close attention to your balance.

➤ *Round and Release – This exercise encourages you to focus on your abdominal muscles and strengthens your abs and back. The focus on tightening and relaxing of muscle groups is good preparation for labor.*
- With your back straight and your ankles crossed, put your hands underneath your knees.
- Breathe in, then breathe out pulling your navel toward your spine as you curl your back into a "C."
- Breathe in and return to the starting position.

➤ *Ankle Exercise – This exercise is good for relaxing your feet and ankles, which can become tired and swollen with the added weight of your baby.*
- To get into position, sit with your back against the wall, your feet raised, and your lower legs supported by a pillow. (Make sure that your feet are in alignment with your legs not pointed in or out.)
- Stretch your feet forward as far as possible without letting your legs come off of the pillow, then point and stretch your toes holding the stretch for a count of five.
- Flex your feet back to their original position and then point and flex rhythmically.
- Circle your ankle five times clockwise, then switch and go counter clockwise.

To find Pilates classes, call local health clubs or check for a Pilates studio in your area. They sometimes offer pre- and postnatal classes. Like any exercise, Pilates may not work for you so if you're uncomfortable with the moves, back off. Now isn't the time to try anything too complicated. Stick with the basics and listen to your body.

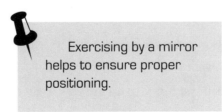
Exercising by a mirror helps to ensure proper positioning.

Yoga

The practice of yoga dates back so far that it is hard to trace it roots, but it is clear that the practice has become part of mainstream western culture in recent decades and a focus on pre-natal and post-partum yoga has become increasingly popular.

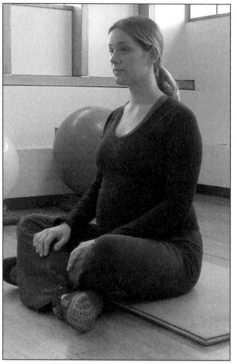

Breathing technique is a key element in yoga.

It is said that the popular Lamaze® technique of breathing and relaxation are rooted in yoga. While yoga has obvious mind-body benefits, it also is known to help pregnant women maintain normal blood pressure, prevent rapid weight gain, and strengthen pelvic floor muscles. The core of yoga is the breathing technique, which brings air slowly through your nose, down to fill your lungs, and out until your stomach is fully compressed. The calm and efficient breathing is an important tool for labor as contractions come and go.

Ann, a mother of two, has been practicing yoga for fifteen years.

"I was in good shape going into childbirth and also doing yoga and dancing helped my body know how to move in childbirth, yoga helped me be flexible and strong and dance helped me hand myself over to the movement more than I think I would have known how to do without having done it. The images from yoga also helped during childbirth, the first time because a friend was actively helping me remember those images, the second time because they were more accessible to me."

After pregnancy, yoga is easy to take back up and its stimulation of blood flow helps invigorate and heal your body. It is also a practice that many women take up with their young children from practicing at home to attending special classes for mother and child.

Some Yoga Poses

► *Standing Mountain – The continuous flow of this exercise warms up your body for other movements.*

- Stand with your feet farther than hip-width part, knees slightly bent and toes pointed straight ahead, and palms touching at "heart center" in front of your chest.
- Close your eyes and breathe deeply.
- Breathe in while sweeping your arms overhead and pointed slightly backward.
- Exhale and stand upright while returning your hands to their starting position at heart center.
- Repeat for 10 full breaths.

► *Squatting – Squatting poses are good everyday practice during pregnancy as they relax and open the pelvis while also strengthening the upper legs. Later in pregnancy you may want to do supported squats using pillows or yoga blocks.*

- Stand facing the back of a chair with your feet slightly farther than hip-width apart and your toes pointed outward.
- Hold onto the chair for balance and support.
- Lower your tailbone toward the floor as if you are going to sit down on a chair.
- Contract your abdominal muscles, lift your chest and relax your shoulders while also finding your balance. Your weight should be resting on your heels.
- Take a deep breath and then exhale pushing into your legs and up to a standing position.

➤ **Full Butterfly** – *This position helps relieve tension from inner thigh muscles and helps tired legs.*

- Sit with legs outstretched.
- Bend your knees and bring the soles of your feet together, keeping the heels as close to the body as possible. Fully relax the inner thighs.
- Clasp the feet with both hands.
- Gently bounce your knees up and down, using your elbows as levers to press the legs down. Do not use any force.
- Repeat up to 20-30 times. Straighten the legs and relax.

The butterfly pose helps relieve inner thigh tension.

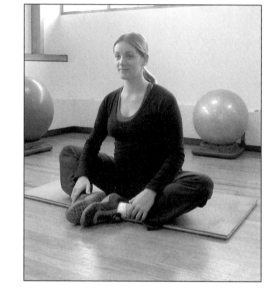

➤ **Cobbler or Tailor pose** – *This pose helps open up the pelvis.*

- Sit up straight with your back against a wall and the soles of your feet touching each other.
- Gently press your knees down and away from each other being careful not to force them apart.
- Stay in the position as long as it is comfortable. (If you are loose jointed, place pillows beneath your knees to avoid overextension of the hips.)

➤ *Seated Pelvic Circles – This movement will be useful in early labor. It may relieve pressure on your back and pelvis and encourage the baby to descend into the pelvis.*

- Sit upright on a stack of pillows with your legs crossed and your hands on your lower belly.
- Move your pelvis in a slow, circular motion, relaxing into the movement.

Samantha, mother of a baby girl, shares her experience practicing and teaching yoga during pregnancy. Samantha has been practicing yoga routinely since 1998. She has a background in Birkram and Iyengar yoga as well as multi-style practices, and has instructed yoga at the University of Vermont and Ben & Jerry's corporate division.

"My yoga practice stayed pretty consistent throughout my pregnancy. Because I have had a daily practice for three years now, my body is aware of the postures. During pregnancy, I practiced vinyasa yoga, which is a flowing sequence coordinated with rhythmic breathing.

For about eight weeks in the early stage of pregnancy I was very sick so I didn't do much of anything. I really had to honor my body and let nature take its course. I did have to modify certain postures to accommodate my belly, but other than that I practiced this style until the day I gave birth.

I did continue to teach during my pregnancy. I had to eliminate some classes because of some fatigue, but I have to say I really didn't face any challenges teaching. I would modify or teach off the mat if I wasn't feeling great.

After those nauseating eight weeks, I felt great. I had good energy and strength and was maintaining a normal weight as my belly grew! I know that practicing yoga throughout my pregnancy kept me fit and grounded.

My labor was ten hours from start to finish. That is really not a long time for a first child. Once the baby was in place, I pushed for half an hour. My hips were definitely open due to my daily practice. My mind was also open due to my practice, so I was able to deliver with minimal drugs.

My daughter and I already practice yoga. She loves the side stretches and the 'heart warm touch,' where I lay one hand on her heart and one hand on my heart for about 5 minutes. It is great bonding."

The benefits of yoga are not only limited to your physical well being. Taking a prenatal yoga class is a great way to meet other pregnant women. By being in a positive, supportive group with other pregnant women, you can get an ongoing emotional boost and stay motivated to continue exercising.

Exercise Ball

An exercise ball, which you may come to know as a "birthing ball" during labor, can have many uses for stretching and strengthening during pregnancy. While most hospitals and birthing centers have the balls on hand to be used for comfortable movement during labor, you can also take your own ball along if you have gotten used to it in the months leading up to the big day.

To prevent slipping, use the ball on a rug or yoga mat or wear shoes to keep your feet in firm position. Twelve to fifteen repetitions are recommended for each exercise.

Exercise balls have become especially popular in the birthing process and in prenatal exercise because sitting on the ball takes the pressure off of your uterus. The ball is essentially a fitness tool that helps you strengthen muscles and improve balance. The exercise ball can also be used for a variety of Pilates movements.

Exercise balls are available at many fitness centers and also can be purchased in sports shops and department stores. They are available in different sizes so be sure to find one that fits your height. Also, follow the inflation instructions as the more you inflate the ball, the harder it will be to balance on.

When you sit on the ball, your knees should be aligned with your hips making a right angle and your feet should be hip-width apart.

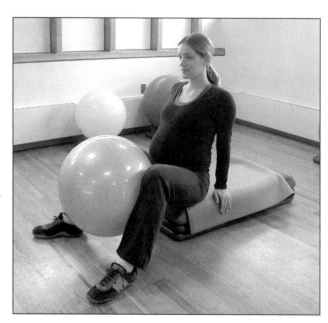

You can use a ball for an abduction squeeze which strengthens the inner thigh muscles. Squeeze in with your knees, hold it for a few seconds, and gently release.

Some Exercise Ball Drills

► *Balance – This is a good exercise to keep doing throughout pregnancy, as it will keep all the torso muscles toned.*

- Sit upright on top of the ball with your arms relaxed by your sides and feet flat on the floor. Be aware of your back, abdominal, and leg muscles, which are keeping you balanced.
- Reach your arms up overhead and squeeze your shoulder blades down and together as you lower your arms to starting position.

Stay centered without moving your torso as you raise and lower your arms.

► *Wall Squat And Back Massage*
- Put the ball between your lower back and the wall.
- Lean back against the ball, and walk your feet out so they're in front of your belly, hip-width apart.
- Place your hands on your thighs and slowly bend your knees into a squat position. Keep your knees and ankles aligned and squat no lower than your hips.
- Then, press gently against the ball and feel it roll up your back.
- Straighten your knees and hips back to a standing position.

► *Belly Breathing*
- Sit comfortably on the ball.
- Breathe in allowing your abdomen to expand.
- Exhale by contracting your abs to force the breath out.
- Work up to completing 20 repetitions to strengthen your abdominal muscles.

Pilates, yoga, and the exercise ball are wonderful exercises to practice during pregnancy. They can help you maintain muscle tone and keep you flexible with little if any impact on your joints. They also help you breathe and relax. These exercises can help you adjust to the physical demands of labor, birth, and motherhood. Combine them with some aerobic activity and you are well on your way to being Fit & Pregnant.

"Exercise really lifts my spirits and helps me feel positive about getting larger." A mother who attended a prenatal aerobics class twice a week during her first pregnancy

Chapter 7

Aerobics

The research and writing of Dr. Kenneth Cooper helped to create the aerobic exercise movement in this country. Aerobic means "using oxygen" which happens every time we perform an exercise such as running, walking, cycling, or aerobic dance. Our body meets the challenge of sustaining physical activity by improving its ability to get oxygen from our lungs to our working muscles. This is what we call cardiovascular fitness. Dr. Cooper's belief in the physical and emotional benefits of aerobic exercise started Americans moving aerobically.

Aerobic dance first gained popularity in the seventies. Jackie Sorenson was one of the early designers of choreographed movements to music. As its popularity grew, new forms evolved: Jazzercise®, low impact, high impact, water aerobics, and bench step aerobics. Today, many women like yourself attend aerobics classes on a regular basis at health clubs, aerobics studios, YWCA's and in your home with videotapes and DVDs.

"Exercise kept me energized," recalls Alane, a mother of two. Prior to pregnancy Alane taught aerobic dance two to four hours a week. She continued to teach until her fifth month when her growing size made it difficult to both instruct the class and perform the workout. Instead, she attended aerobics 1 to 2 hours a week and began a prenatal water fitness program once a week. She continued low impact aerobics, making adjustments for back discomfort by avoiding certain floor exercises, until the eighth month. "I was concerned about maintaining fitness and tone during pregnancy, but toward the end, I found I concentrated more on flexibility than aerobic exercise."

Alane's first labor lasted 19 hours which surprised her. She thought being fit would make her labor easier.

Women join aerobics classes for many reasons. "Exercise helps keep me fit and toned and gives me an energy boost," says Karen, a mother of two. She attends an aerobics class three times a week at a local health club. For many women, aerobics is a fun way to get exercise. There's class camaraderie, the diversion of music and an enthusiastic instructor to motivate you and lead you through the workout. By attending a well-designed aerobics class at least three times a week, you will improve your cardiovascular fitness and flexibility, strengthen and tone your muscles and leave your workouts with a relaxed, yet invigorated feeling. (See Chapter 10 for water aerobics.)

What Makes A Good Aerobics Class?

► *The Instructor*

Your instructor should be knowledgeable, enthusiastic, and preferably certified. There are several organizations which offer certification including The Aerobics and Fitness Association of America (AFAA), The American Council on Exercise (ACE), and the American College of Sports Medicine (ACSM). The instructor has the responsibility of conducting a safe class and monitoring the intensity of the workout during the aerobic phase of the class.

► *The Class*

All classes, (low impact, high impact and bench step aerobics) generally follow a similar format. Low impact classes are less stressful to your joints by keeping leg and foot motions low to the ground. One foot remains on the floor at all times. High impact includes more jumping and hopping while bench step aerobics incorporates choreographed stepping movements on and off a platform. Each of these classes starts with a warm-up/stretching phase which slowly warms up all of your major muscle groups. Warmed, flexible muscles are less prone to injury. Your pulse rate slowly rises in preparation for the work ahead.

> *"Stretching helps promote muscle balance and flexibility and prevents muscle soreness. Don't be tempted to skip it."* Kathryn, an aerobics instructor, who emphasizes the importance of the stretching portion of the class

The cardiovascular phase is usually 20 to 60 minutes of choreographed arm and leg movements which raises your heart rate. Periodically checking your pulse lets you know how you are progressing but remember that pulse rate is not a reliable indicator of workout intensity during pregnancy. However, as you warm up, you will be "utilizing oxygen" more efficiently and becoming more fit. You gradually slow your movements down and lower your pulse rate as you begin the strength and toning phase.

This workout phase targets specific muscle groups to build strength and improve tone for both your upper and lower body. Hand-held weights or stretch bands can add resistance to this part of the workout. When using weights or stretch bands, avoid holding your breath. Exhale during the contraction of the muscle and inhale during the release. We'll cover this in more detail in the next chapter.

The cool down phase incorporates slow, rhythmic movements to lower your heart rate and prevent blood from pooling in your extremities. This is followed by stretching all your major muscle groups while breathing slowly and deeply.

► *The Facility*

Try to find a facility with an aerobics room large enough to accommodate all participants. Look for wooden or tightly carpeted floor surfaces (no concrete) as well as air-conditioning and good ventilation. Make sure that there are drinking water and bathroom facilities nearby. The facility should have mirrors to help check for correct body positions and to increase the visibility of the instructor. Good acoustics and an adequate sound system are also important considerations.

"I felt that it was the best thing for me and my baby," Karen, a thirty one year old mother of two said when she described the program of low impact aerobics, Stairmaster™ and walking she used during her last pregnancy. During the last two months before delivery, she did more walking due to discomfort from varicose veins. Her second baby was a vaginal delivery after a prior Cesarean section (VBAC). She attributes her stamina during labor and delivery to her exercise program during pregnancy.

Aerobics For Two

The primary goal of any prenatal fitness program is the safety of you and your fetus. Before you became pregnant, your exercise goals might have been to stay trim and toned and perhaps to lose weight. Routines you may have used then, the intense, vigorous workouts designed to reduce weight, are not safe now that you are pregnant. Most studies agree that prenatal exercise programs should be low impact and moderate intensity. Let's look at how you can still use aerobics to stay fit.

A well-designed prenatal aerobics class takes into account your body's tremendous physical changes can offer many benefits during your pregnancy. You can reduce backache, swelling, pelvic pressure, excessive weight gain, and fatigue. You can maintain your aerobic fitness and muscular strength and flexibility. An active, moving body also enhances self-esteem and builds self-confidence.

A certified instructor who is trained in the physiology, anatomy and biomechanics of pregnancy should teach the prenatal aerobics class. Classes should be individualized and follow the current 2002 ACOG guidelines for exercise in pregnancy (see Chapter 3). Before starting a class, discuss your plans with your health care provider who is familiar with your fitness level, medical history, and the health of your pregnancy.

Specialized classes for pregnant women provide closer individual monitoring in a supportive environment. You can discuss pregnancy-related topics and experiences shared by the group.

"I am at the end of my eighth month and definitely feel stronger and more confident about my pregnancy because of the prenatal aerobics class. I have gained weight in the right places and not the wrong ones." Diane, during her first pregnancy.

General Guidelines For Prenatal Aerobics

As mentioned previously, you need to discuss your exercise plans with your health care provider. Let your instructor know of any special concerns or recent developments in your pregnancy. Eat a light snack about an hour before class. Drink plenty of fluids and bring your water bottle to class. Remember, you sweat more in pregnancy so dress in light, breathable clothing. Layering is a good idea so you can peel off as you warm up. Avoid exercising in hot, humid conditions or if you have a fever. Wear a panty liner if you have vaginal discharge or problems with leaking urine. A good supportive bra is important. Shoes designed for aerobics are best. Listen to your body. Exercise according to how you feel and not how you think you should be exercising.

Your changing body requires modification of exercises to avoid injury or discomfort. The hormones of pregnancy make your joints and ligaments more relaxed and vulnerable to strain or sprains. Your added weight changes your posture causing you to lean forward slightly. In turn, this shift in your center of gravity causes some muscles in your body to relax and others to tighten. A prenatal aerobics class must modify certain exercises, especially to those areas of your body under "mechanical stress" such as your abdomen, pelvis, back and hips.

Abdominal Exercise Modifications

You should modify abdominal exercises after the fourth month to avoid putting direct pressure on the abdominal muscles. For example, you can do abdominal curl-ups in a semirecumbent position with knees rolled to the side. Crossing your arms over your abdomen can provide additional support to the abdominal wall. Also, you should keep in mind that exercising from the supine position (flat on your back) causes the weight of your uterus to compress the vena cava, a large vein that returns blood from your lower body to your heart. This can cause a drop in blood pressure (supine hypotension) making you feel dizzy or faint.

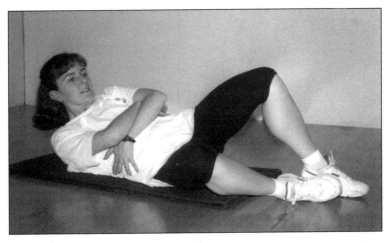

After your fourth month, modify abdominal exercises to avoid putting direct pressure on your abdominal muscles.

Diastasis recti is the complete or partial separation of the rectus abdominis muscle. Most common in the third trimester of pregnancy, it is caused by weak abdominal muscles, a big baby, obesity, heredity, and other factors. You can measure the degree of separation. Ask your health provider to teach you how to check for this. Avoid abdominal work if there is a separation of these muscles.

Pelvic Exercise Modifications

The pelvic floor refers to the muscles and fascia that support your pelvic organs, the bladder, uterus, and rectum. During pregnancy, leaking of urine can be a sign of weakness in these muscles. The Kegel exercise is an isometric contraction of these muscles. You can learn this by trying to hold your flow of urine midstream. Once you are able to effectively isolate these muscles, you can incorporate Kegels into abdominal and buttocks exercises. I remind women to do Kegel exercises at every stoplight while driving. As you'll read later, it is good to continue Kegels after pregnancy. One plan is to Kegel while breastfeeding.

Large ligaments help support your expanding uterus. The constant stretching of these ligaments can cause irritation, especially with sudden movements. Again, modified abdominal exercises will reduce discomfort. Keep your knee and hip joints slightly bent while doing hip abductions (leg moving outward) and hip adductions (leg moving inward). Instead of using the "all fours" position for buttocks exercises, try standing for working these muscles. Move slowly from side to side and practice proper body mechanics by using your arms when rising from the floor.

Backaches

The weight of your uterus pulls your pelvis forward causing you to curve your lower back, round your shoulders, and lean your head forward. This postural change causes lower backache. Exercises should focus on strengthening your back, hip and abdominal muscles as well as stretching and relaxing the back, shoulders and neck. The cat stretch is an easy back stretch to do. Get on all fours (hands and knees) and round your back toward the ceiling as you exhale. Inhale as you lower your back to a flat position. The cat stretch can also relieve strain to the pelvic ligaments.

Muscle Cramps

You can trigger muscle cramps in your thighs or calves by pointing your toes during a routine. They are also common at night when a pain suddenly awakens you in your calf muscle. Relief will come by stretching the muscle and holding it until the cramp subsides. Straighten your knee for a hamstring cramp and dorsiflex your foot (pull back the toes) for a calf cramp.

Warm Up Before Bed
If you are having nighttime muscle cramps, do a five minute leg warm-up before bed. Do some ankle rolls and any circulation enhancing movement

Prenatal Class Format

Let's talk about a prenatal class format designed for the "two" of you.

► *Warm-up*

Gentle stretching and range of motion exercises helps get your joints, ligaments and muscles ready for movement. Focus attention on your vulnerable areas: your pelvic ligaments, your lower back and your hips. Stretch to the point of mild tension, not pain. Breathe in and out slowly. Avoid holding your breath.

► *Aerobics (non-impact)*

Avoid bouncy, jerky movements and sudden changes in direction. Movements should be smooth and controlled. Pay attention to good posture. Keep your legs moving while standing to avoid pooling of blood. The intensity of your workout should be "somewhat hard," or 12 to 14 on the RPE scale (See Chapter 3.) Be sure to drink water at frequent intervals. Avoid overheating. Stop if you feel any pain or discomfort.

► *Short Cooldown*

Slow your heart rate down with easy rhythmic leg movements and gentle stretches. It's time to replace some fluids and empty your bladder before starting the body work.

► *Body Work (muscular strength and flexibility)*

You work the upper and lower body plus abdominals using smooth and controlled movements. Remember to exhale during the contraction of muscles and inhale during the release. Avoid the supine position for abdominals. Practice good body alignment and body mechanics when changing position.

► *Final Cooldown*

Combine gentle stretching and relaxation with slow deep breathing. Your pulse rate should be back to normal before you leave class, feeling refreshed and invigorated.

> *"I always felt great after class. I had more energy and felt positive," remarks Julie about her prenatal aerobics class.*

Moms In Motion

Sara Kooperman, JD, now the CEO of SCW Fitness Education, the largest producer of fitness instructor training videos in the world, designed Moms in Motion, a prenatal exercise program offered at St. Joseph's Healthcare Hospital in Michigan. The program helps pregnant women safely exercise during pregnancy, taking into account the tremendous body changes in pregnancy. The following are some of Moms In Motion guidelines for a safe fitness program in pregnancy.

Prior to enrolling in class, all of the students obtain a note of approval from their health care provider. Students are advised to eat a light snack one to two hours before class and to bring a water bottle and towel for floor work. The instructor advises students to exercise at their own level and to listen to any signals their body might be sending during the workout. The class avoids high impact and power moves (sudden jumps or thrusts) as well as exercises using rubber bands around the ankles. (Some swelling in pregnancy is common so this might cause trauma to the tissue as well as impair circulation.) Likewise, the class avoids any exercises with the head below the heart. (In this position, your expanded blood volume can cause you to feel faint.) Kegel exercises are included in every class to strengthen the pelvic floor muscles. Each student is observed and offered pointers for modifying exercises during each trimester. Time is spent in class talking about pregnancy-related issues like hormonal changes, breast and bottle-feeding, baby equipment and other topics.

> *"Participating in Moms In Motion gave me more energy and I had an opportunity to meet other pregnant women. It was a lot of fun."* Alison, former program participant

What if a prenatal aerobics isn't available where you live? One option is to purchase a prenatal exercise videotape or DVD. Make sure that the material follows the ACOG guidelines and that you take the same precautions as you would if you were participating in an aerobics class. Be sure to exercise in a cool room and drink plenty of fluids.

Another option is to integrate into a regular aerobics class. Discuss this plan with your health care provider. A low impact aerobics class, or bench step class using the platform only with no risers, is safest. Let the instructor know that you are pregnant and closely follow all of the exercise guidelines in pregnancy. Do not try to "keep up" with the class. Instead, exercise at your own pace, paying attention to any signs of discomfort or strain. You may need to eliminate parts of the workout or shorten it all together.

When To Stop?

You need to stop exercising if you feel any of the following symptoms: Increased uterine contractions, decreased fetal movements, vaginal bleeding, leaking of amniotic fluid, dizziness or faintness, shortness of breath, palpitations, persistent nausea or vomiting, back pain or hip pain, or difficulty walking.

Remember, there's a silent passenger on board, so you need to tune into any signals your body might be sending during your aerobics program. Here is an example of one woman who modified her aerobics routine during pregnancy:

Kathy, a mother of three and former teacher, participated in gymnastics from age seven to thirteen and then competed in diving during high school. During college she started attending aerobics classes on a regular basis. While pregnant with her first two children, she was able to participate in low impact aerobics three times a week, avoiding abdominals after her fourth month. In her third pregnancy, she attended a bench step class, using the platform without risers. She stopped using any hand weights and did easy arm movements. Kathy felt most comfortable in Spandex shorts and a baggy T-shirt.

In each of her pregnancies, she turned to swimming during the last two months because of pelvic pressure and varicose veins. Kathy felt great in the water. With her first pregnancy, because she was not yet a proficient swimmer, she held a kickboard under her chest and kicked her way up and down the lap lanes. She swam until delivery without any major problems. Occasionally, when climbing out of the pool, she would feel the "pull of gravity" on her abdomen. After a few seconds, she adjusted to being out of the buoyant water environment. Kathy monitored herself carefully during all of her pregnancies and cut back or modified according to how she felt. "I really enjoyed exercising. I felt it helped me maintain my shape as much as possible as well as allowed me time to clear my head." All of Kathy's babies were delivered vaginally and weighed between 7 and 7 3/4 pounds.

Aerobics can strengthen your heart and lungs and help maintain muscle tone during your pregnancy. Choose exercises that are low impact (no high kicks and leaps), and keep one foot on the ground at all times to minimize stress on your joints — you should be able to continue aerobics through most of your pregnancy.

"I always listened to my body and was extremely cautious. I stopped if anything felt sore or uncomfortable. My husband was very supportive as was everyone else at the fitness center." Weight lifter and first time mother

Chapter 8

Weight Training

Walk into any health club and you will see and hear the impact of the weight training industry. The clank of weights and the whirl of cables and pulleys signal that everybody's "using it" so they don't "lose it." There are many good reasons why you too should include weight training in your exercise program. Besides getting stronger, which can enhance athletic performance, you can ward off injuries, build stronger bones, boost your metabolism, feel better about yourself and look great in the process. No wonder the industry is booming!

Weight training is progressive resistance exercise. Free weights (dumbbells and barbells) and exercise machines provide the resistance to the muscles you are working. Resistance stimulates muscle growth as well as improving muscle strength and endurance. You should develop a weight training program that is based on completing certain exercises grouped together by repetitions and sets. Repetitions (reps) are the number of times you do an exercise and sets are the number of groupings of repetitions. Before we look at pregnancy-specific weight training, let's review the basics of a weight training program.

Principles Of Weight Training

You should design an individualized weight training program that will meet your goals. Perhaps your goal is to improve your muscular endurance, or maybe it is to build overall strength, or even more likely, to trim and tone as you lose weight. Weight training, when coupled with aerobic exercise and proper diet, can help with weight loss. Aerobic exercise burns calories while lifting weights builds muscles. Bigger muscles burn calories more efficiently so it's like cranking up your metabolism. You can achieve all of these goals with a well designed, yet simple, weight training program.

Two basic principles, specificity and overload, form the foundation of weight training. Specificity means that you target certain muscle groups in your workout. For

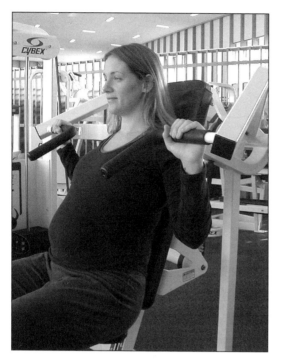

Some women may want to improve their upper body strength.

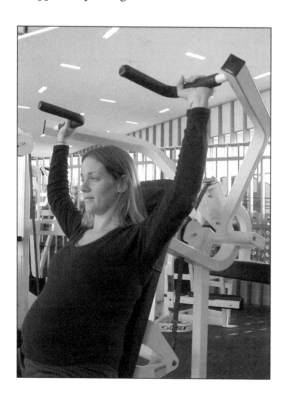

example, some women may want to improve their upper body strength. If you are a runner, there's a good chance that you have neglected your upper body strength. A strong upper body helps you maintain good posture, run more efficiently and keep your form. By having a stronger upper body, you'll expend less energy and run farther and faster. Cyclists will want to focus more on strengthening their legs and cross country skiers want both upper and lower body strength. One thing to keep in mind is this: a strong upper body is every mother's blessing — as you struggle to carry your baby, diaper bag and groceries — all at one time.

The overload principle requires you to progressively increase the intensity of your workout over time in a set pattern. You will do this over a period of weeks and months. Muscles, to get stronger, need to be challenged by slowly increasing the resistance, the number of repetitions, and the rate of work. Using both the specificity and overload concepts, you design a program of weight training which determines the load (amount of weight), the number of reps and sets and the recovery period between the sets.

Trainers, available through health clubs, can help you design your program using these principles. Make sure the person you are working with is qualified and certified by one of these organizations — NSCA (National Strength and Conditioning Association), ACE (American Council on Exercise), ACSM (American College of Sports Medicine). For further information on their web sites, see the Resource Section.

Lifting Fundamentals And Equipment

Before discussing lifting techniques, let's talk about the importance of a warm-up before your workout and a cooldown afterwards. To avoid injury and help your muscles recover, warm-up with 10 to 15 minutes of brisk walking, jogging, or stationary cycling followed by stretching. This kind of warm-up prepares your muscles and joints for the work ahead. Be sure to include stretches for the chest, shoulders, arms, back, and large muscle groups (hamstrings, quadriceps and calves). Don't forget to cool down (easy jogging, walking) and stretch after your workout to prevent muscle soreness. (See Chapter 5 for more information.)

Weight Training Tips
- Adjust levers and seats to comfortable positions. (These may change during your pregnancy.)
- Avoid bouncing the weight stacks.
- Perform each exercise slowly and with control, using a full range of motion.
- Load the bars evenly.
- Properly lock the barbells and dumbbells — don't assume the person ahead of you did.
- Be aware of other lifters around you — pay attention!
- Replace and store the equipment you use.

Weight training machines are generally safer than free weights. You don't have to worry about weights falling on you nor do you need the help of a "spotter," someone who assists you in performing a particular lift. Become familiar with the machines at your facility. If you are not sure about a particular machine — ask.

► Technique

Proper technique is very important whether you are using free weights or weight machines. You cannot only avoid injuries to muscles, tendons, and bones, you can get better results.

► Correct Lifting

Use a light grip — not a "death" grip. The focus of your energy should be on the muscles you are working rather than your hands. Lift from a stable position. Keep the weight close to your body.

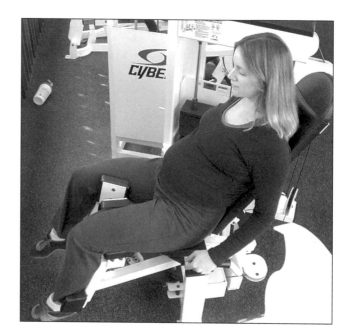

Hip abductor machines will build strength in your hips that will help you overcome postural changes during your pregnancy.

► Breathing

Whether using weight machines or free weights, you always want to breathe out (exhale) during the lifting or exertion phase and breathe in (inhale) during the recovery or lowering phase. During pregnancy, avoid the Valsalva maneuver (holding your breath while lifting or moving a weight). Holding your breath while lifting can raise your blood pressure and decrease blood flow to the uterus.

► Spotters

Some lifts require spotters, someone who is ready to assist you as you perform lifts like the bench press. During your pregnancy it is best to avoid the lifts that require a spotter. There are safer alternative exercises you can do with weight machines.

I am assuming that you have worked with a trainer to set up a weight training program and that you have already determined your training loads for each exercise. A training load is a set weight that allows you to do up to 12 reps (repetitions) of that particular exercise. With each rep you use slow controlled movements, a full range of motion, and proper breathing techniques. (Remember to exhale with the lift, inhale with the recovery.) For best results, try to weight train two to three days a week, with a recovery day after each session. Your program should work all the muscle groups — chest, arms, shoulders, back, thighs and abdomen. Try to:

1. Work all the large muscles first.
2. Alternate push with pull exercises.
3. Alternate upper body with lower body exercises.
4. Work opposing muscle groups i.e., biceps/triceps, quads/hamstrings, etc.

Tailor your program around the training loads, the number of reps (usually 8-12), the number of sets (the times you perform the block of reps — usually 2 to 3 sets), and the rest periods between each set. As you get stronger, you can increase the training loads.

If you are pressed for time, you can do split routines which allows you to work for a shorter period of time on specific body parts on different days. For example, in a four day per week program, two workouts would focus on your upper body (chest, shoulders, triceps, biceps, upper abdominal, upper back) and the other two workouts would concentrate on your lower body (legs, lower back, lower abdominal).

Pregnancy Weight Training

Most of you will find that you can continue weight training during your pregnancy as long as you modify your routine and take some basic precautions. Stick with weight machines unless you are experienced with free weights.

Use slow, controlled movements to lift weights to avoid injuring your joints that are loosened during pregnancy. Work with lighter weights than you normally do and to compensate for the lower weight, you can do more repetitions. (1 to 2 sets of 12 to 15 reps). Many exercise centers have exercise bands — stretchy, rubber bands which are also available from sporting good stores. Stretch bands don't put as much sudden pressure on the muscles, ligaments, or joints, but still provide the muscle and ligament toning that dumbbells do. As with any exercise activity, be sure to consult with your health care provider if there are any special concerns about your pregnancy or general health.

Now, more than ever, you need to practice good technique and follow all the lifting fundamentals.

Here are some important points to consider.

► *Warm-up/Cooldown*

As mentioned earlier, pregnancy relaxes your joints and ligaments. Proper warm-up and cooldown will prevent injury. Allow time for both.

► *Fluids*

Carry your water bottle with you on your circuit and drink often.

► *Clothing*

Wear comfortable clothing. A large T-shirt over cycling-style shorts or tights works well. Stay cool. Don't overdress. Supportive running or aerobic shoes work fine.

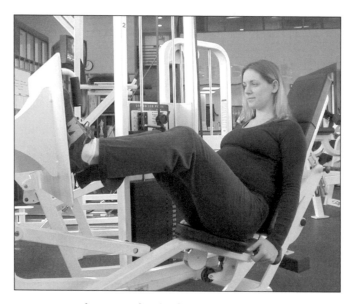

Leg presses are a good exercise for the first trimester. They give you a good workout and keep your lower abdominals tight to protect your back.

Exercises To Avoid

After the first trimester, you should avoid exercises which require you to lie on your back (supine position) or stomach. You can still work these muscles in a more upright position. For example, for the chest, instead of the free weight bench press or dumbbell flys, you can substitute the bent arm fly using a "pec dec" chest machine. This machine can approximate the fly movement and works your pectoral (chest) muscles. For your back, use resistance bands or the seated rowing exercise instead of the barbell bent-over row exercise.

Beginning in the second trimester, avoid lifting weights while standing. Avoid lying on a bench to lift weights or assuming any position that leaves your abdomen vulnerable to a falling weight.

Avoid power lifting and quick-lift exercises. Power lifting is a sport that develops maximum strength using specific lifts. Quick-lifts require explosive movements. Do neither of these techniques during your pregnancy. If you body build, discuss this with your health provider.

Practice Safe Lifting Techniques

As your pregnancy continues and you get bigger, your center of gravity will shift. Pay attention to your body position as you perform your exercise circuit. Use good body mechanics as you load weight machines with weights. Your lower back is vulnerable to injury as well as joints and ligaments. Working with a friend or partner is fun. Then, you can converse as you lift, which helps keep your heart rate down, and you will have someone to observe your technique. Your partner can also remind you to breathe correctly — to exhale with the lift, inhale on recovery.

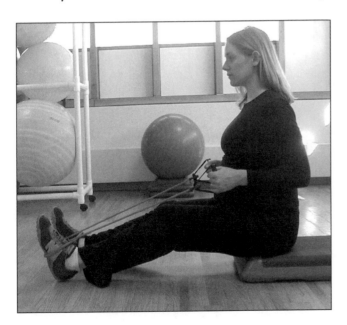

Instead of bent rows with a barbell, do a seated row with exercise bands.

Modify Modify Modify

As your body changes over the next nine months, so will your weight training program. Switch to lighter weights and moderate repetitions. Extend your recovery phase in-between exercises. Always work under the supervision of your health care provider and a trained fitness instructor. Listen to your body. You are weight training to maintain tone and fitness — not to re-sculpture your body or train for power lifting. Stop if you feel faint, short of breath, or experience any pain or bleeding.

Shannon's Program

During high school Shannon played volleyball and softball and ran cross-country. When she entered college, she began weight training to improve her overall strength and endurance. Her studies in exercise science helped her to design a program to achieve these goals. As her fitness and strength improved, so did her commitment to her weight training program. When she finished college she took a position as a fitness coordinator at a university fitness and wellness center. At this point, her program consisted of twenty minutes of aerobic exercise (Stairmaster) followed by 1 to 1.5 hours of weight training three to six days a week using both free weights and weight machines.

When Shannon learned she was pregnant, she wanted to continue her program with some modifications. At her first prenatal visit, accompanied by her husband, she discussed her current fitness program with her health care provider. Together, they agreed that the health of her pregnancy was the number one priority and that her new fitness goal was to maintain her fitness and not to improve on strength and endurance. Shannon and her health provider reviewed the exercise guidelines for pregnancy. (See Chapter 3).

Her program remained the same during her first trimester though now she made sure she ate a light snack an hour before her workout and drank plenty of water. Plagued by some nausea and fatigue, she found that exercising helped relieve these symptoms. By the second trimester she eliminated any lifting on her back or stomach and cut back on her workouts. Shannon gradually decreased the weights and increased the reps to the 12 to 15 range.

By the time Shannon went into labor she had gained about 24 pounds. During her labor, the fetus' heart rate pattern was showing signs of distress. A healthy baby boy, "Cyrus," was delivered by Cesarean section and weighed in at nine pounds, one ounce.

"I think being in shape helped give me the stamina to tolerate labor better, and it certainly helped me with recovery after the surgery. I was slowly able to get back to my program." Shannon

Shannon's story is a good lesson: exercise does not guarantee the elimination of complications during pregnancy and delivery. Yet it is important to keep in mind that you and your baby are still ahead of the game in spite of one or two setbacks.

"In my first trimester, I ran as often as I could despite bouts of morning sickness and pelvic pressure. I knew that I was not going to be one of those women with a tiny, pregnant belly who runs practically up until her due date. So I ran and ran and ran until I had to switch to walking (which didn't feel like exercise) and swimming and cross country skiing, which were low-impact alternatives that I could handle for the duration of my pregnancies." Runner and mother of two

Chapter 9

Running, Walking, Hiking

Running

The beauty of running is its simplicity. Strap on a pair of running shoes, find a road or trail, and you are ready for an invigorating cardiovascular workout. When running outdoors, it's fun to treat your senses to the sights, smells and sounds of your route, letting the fresh mown grass, the colorful leaves, or the crunching snow remind you of the changing seasons. Running is a time-efficient aerobic activity. You can squeeze a workout into a lunch hour, go out before breakfast, or tag a run on at the end of the day. Even with a busy schedule, you can usually find time for a run — something to keep in mind, especially after you have the baby and time is precious.

If you already run, you will likely want to continue it during pregnancy. In general, running is a safe activity that many pregnant women continue, with modification, throughout pregnancy. If you've never run before, now is not the time to start. If you are a seasoned runner, enjoy the journey ahead, but stay open to incorporating other sorts of exercise activities into your schedule.

The classic study on running and pregnancy was done in the early 1980's by the Melpomene Institute, a non-profit organization which publishes research and educational material on fitness and health for girls and women. One hundred ninety-five women, whose average age was 29.1 years, were studied. Three months before conception they were averaging 24.8 miles per week. 80.3% of the women delivered vaginally while 19.7% had Cesarean sections. The average birth weight was seven pounds, six ounces. All the infants were born healthy and survived the neonatal period. This report and others on pregnant runners are reassuring but researchers warned that the results do not support racing, speed work, or vigorous long runs. You can continue to run during pregnancy as long as you follow some special guidelines.

Elaine Cooper, writing in *Australian Runner and Athlete*, describes running during early pregnancy.

> *"The first trimester may bring few obvious changes to the outside observer but on the inside it's a hotbed of activity. From about the time the zygote latches onto the lining of the uterus (one week post conception), the runner begins to notice changes that become more and more obvious. Your capacity to cope with these changes during running can vary dramatically according to your pre-pregnancy fitness level, severity of symptoms, psychological attitude, level of support and other stresses (e.g.. work, other children, study).*
>
> *Nausea and fatigue can be two major drawbacks, although their severity and duration may vary remarkably in each woman and in each of her pregnancies. Low blood sugar tends to aggravate these conditions. Try eating little and often. Complex carbohydrates and sufficient protein seem to help. Dieting will aggravate the situation, not to mention the effects it could have on the developing fetus. Running can often ease the nausea. Persevere! While daytime naps are an impossible luxury for most, try to go to bed earlier. Otherwise you'll find running becomes progressively more difficult and you will too.*
>
> *It is around this time you'll notice breathlessness while running, even at a slow pace. The high levels of progesterone supposedly cause a heightened sensitivity to CO_2, resulting in an increased breathing rate. If you're unaware of being pregnant and still racing hard you may notice your lactic tolerance has 'gone out the door'. Middle distance runners relying on a kick in the final lap can forget it. That top gear can vanish quickly."*

Starting The Run

If you're the type who laces up your shoes and then bounds out the door without stretching, change your ways! Now that you're carrying a future runner, you need to take some extra precautions. More than ever, proper stretching both before and after running, will help prevent injuries. Relaxin, the hormone that relaxes your ligaments, is working throughout pregnancy. Loose joints and ligaments make you more vulnerable to injury so concentrate on stretches for your large muscles ... hamstrings, quadriceps, calf muscles, Achilles and lower back muscles. Gentle, easy stretching is best. (See Chapter 5 for specific stretches and cool downs.) Sip some water as you stretch. Listening to some music may help cut the boredom and encourage you to warm up adequately. Hit the bathroom one last time and start out slowly.

Follow a few simple rules to make your run more enjoyable and safer. First, if you're running alone, let someone know your route and the approximate time you'll be back. I suggest that you run with a buddy — it is safer and keeps your workout intensity at the "talk test" level. (You should be able to carry on a conversation as you run.) Second, carry spare change in case you need to make an emergency phone call and always carry some form of identification as well. Third, wear reflective clothing or vests at dawn or dusk or whenever the visibility is low. Finally, leave your iPod® at home. Your attention needs to be on you and the road.

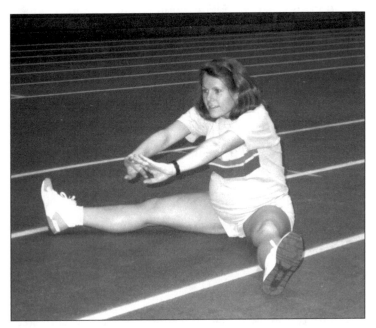

Now, more than ever, proper stretching both before and after running, will help prevent injuries.

Listen To Your Body

You will need to modify the intensity, frequency, and speed of your runs. Remember, you are running to maintain your fitness, not to train. Slow down — don't push your pace, and don't push your distance. Back off running a preset course if you just don't feel like doing it.

Stop and walk if you feel Braxton Hicks contractions (rhythmic tightenings of the lower abdomen) or ligament pains. At seven months, I sometimes felt Braxton Hicks contractions during the first few minutes of a run. I would stop and walk for a few minutes and then, when the contractions stopped, start up again slowly.

Stop if you feel pain, persistent contractions, leakage of fluid, fatigue, dizziness, or any other medical problem.

Where To Run?

Most of you are probably road rats and have several favorite running routes. During pregnancy, you can probably still run most of them if you keep several things in mind:

- Pick a route with a phone and bathroom facility nearby.
- Stay off roads with rough, uneven pavement. You don't want to spend most of your concentration and energy dodging potholes and wobbling along on narrow, fractured road shoulders.
- Skip the routes with steep hills. Uphills may push your intensity level too high. Running downhill puts a lot of stress on your knees and can, due to your additional weight and relaxed joints, lead to knee injuries.

Running on an outdoor track may sound boring to some of you and painfully familiar to others. But, when you're pregnant, you will find the overall the smooth, softer surface kinder to your changing body — and there are usually bathrooms nearby.

Weather conditions will also determine where you run. Snow and ice can make running extremely dangerous — even more so when you are a little top heavy with your pregnancy. Winters in Central New York where I used to live are notorious for persistent snow, and we get used to running on snow-covered roads and sidewalks. Hours before a major record snow storm, I saw our neighbor, nine months pregnant, "jogging" in nearly a foot of snow. When I talked to her later, she admitted that it would have been safer to bag the run and do an indoor workout. When the weather is lousy, move your workout inside. If you have use of an indoor track — great! Other options are a stationary bike, a treadmill, a NordicTrack,® or an aerobics DVD.

What To Wear?

Early in pregnancy, your regular running attire will work fine. As your abdomen begins to expand, you will need clothes that provide comfort and support.

First, let's look at comfort. Wear running gear that is comfortable and doesn't bind. Finally, a good use for all those large race T-shirts! Spandex cycling shorts or tights will stretch as you grow. You may like the added snugness and longer lengths. I know I did.

During the last few months of my pregnancy, I liked wearing a prenatal abdominal support. Even though I was not carrying the pregnancy low, the added support to my lower abdomen felt good. Abdominal support gear comes in different styles and sizes.

If you have varicose veins, running in maternity support hose offers some additional support. As I mentioned in Chapter 2, sport bras or supportive bras with wide adjustable straps are more comfortable for running.

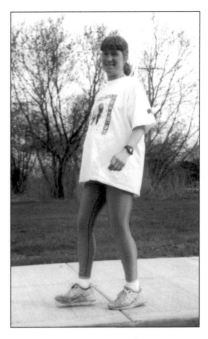

Wear running gear that is comfortable and doesn't bind.

Dress for the weather. Wear light loose fitting clothing in warmer weather. As we noted in Chapter 3, staying cool is important. Avoid running in hazy, hot and humid weather. In cooler weather, dress in layers. You may find that you sweat more when pregnant so check out the new moisture wicking fabrics which will help keep you drier. Protect your extremities when running in the cold. Wear a hat to avoid heat loss off your head as well as warm mittens and gloves. When it's cold, overdress. You can always peel off layers as you go along.

"*The clothing I wore to run during my pregnancy was my husband's shorts and T-shirts — anything with a loose waistband. It's a problem, when you reach that stage where your shorts slide off your stomach and end up around your hips and want to keep going, especially in the last couple of months.*" Elaine Cooper, mother of four

Shoes

Let's take a look at your shoes. You know your feet better than anyone, so the brand and model you're running in now probably works fine. During your pregnancy however, you need to consider a few things about your feet and your running shoes.

Your feet will be supporting a lot more of you in the next nine months. Normally, when running, you land with an impact three times your body weight. Your feet, specifically your heels, will be bearing the brunt of the impact. Put your lighter racing flats away for now. You'll need a shoe with at least 3/4 inch cushioning in the heel. Expect your feet to swell, which can increase your shoe size by a half size. Compensate by wearing a shoe with a wide toe box. Shop for a new pair of running shoes in the afternoon when your feet are apt to be swollen. Buy what feels comfortable. While you are at it, pick up a pair of lace locks — instead of lacing your shoes, you slide the laces through a small plastic device that secures the lace. It beats bending over and tying laces.

The socks you wear should be smooth fitting and conform to your feet. Swelling and sweating — the woes of "pregnant feet" — will feel better in light, synthetic materials that wick away moisture and prevent blisters.

"As soon as I go out to run, it's strange, but it [nausea] is almost immediately gone." An elite runner

Running In Early Pregnancy

You may experience bouts of nausea and fatigue the first few months. Several runners that I interviewed found that running in the morning helped. One runner noted: "After my morning run, my morning sickness always went away."

Try running outdoors if you normally run on an indoor track. The fresh air may help. If you find yourself losing weight from vomiting, cut back your running or stop until you are gaining adequate weight. Talk to your health provider about it.

Fatigue can be perplexing these first few months. As an active woman, you are used to feeling energetic most of the time. Before pregnancy, if you felt sluggish, you probably went out for a run to regain some vigor. Now you may be more inclined to curl up for a nap. The fatigue of early pregnancy can feel as if you're under the influence of a sleeping pill. One woman said, "I felt like I could sleep all day even after an eight hour sleep."

Schedule your run at a time of day when you feel least tired. Don't push it. It can be frustrating — in your mind, you know that running will probably make you feel better, but your body is saying "doze." If running seems too much for today, substitute a brisk walk, a few laps in the pool, or spinning on a stationary bike. Be flexible and patient. The advice to remember is: "This too shall pass."

Linda, a thirty-four year old mother of two, maintained a running schedule during her pregnancies averaging about thirty to thirty-five miles a week. In the first and second trimesters, she ran the same distance but slowed her pace. During the third trimester she ran half as much and supplemented by walking. The added weight and winter conditions made it difficult to continue running the same distance. Linda, like many women I spoke with, felt positive about feeling "fit" during her pregnancies and benefited from the stress reduction of daily exercise.

As mentioned earlier, running with tender swollen breasts is uncomfortable. "It was the least pleasant pregnancy change for me," recalled an elite runner. Buy a good supportive bra with wide adjustable straps or a sports bra. As weeks go by, you may need to move up to a larger size.

Urinary frequency, one of the early signs of pregnancy, is a challenge. (It also returns later in pregnancy because of the added weight and pressure on your bladder.) For running, you need to devise some strategic plans. Don't cut back on your fluids ... you need to stay well hydrated. Plan your runs around a bathroom stop. A twice-around loop that includes a "pit stop" is one option. Consider wearing a panty liner just in case.

As you can see, it's important to tailor your running to how you feel and the health of your pregnancy these first few months. Be sure to immediately stop any racing, speed work, or vigorous long runs once you learn that you are pregnant. Keep your workouts in the "somewhat hard range" in the Rate of Perceived Exertion scale. (See Chapter 3)

Sue is a competitive runner who has competed in triathlons, duathlons, and running races. She has coached high school track and cross country, has served as a personal coach for local runners, and has been involved with many running camps. The mother of two girls, Sue shares her training regimen during pregnancy and how it varied considerably with each pregnancy.

> *"I was able to run throughout my first pregnancy and actually did a five mile race about one month prior to my delivery. I ran in other races, although I would not consider it racing. I really tried to pace myself in the races, feeling comfortable starting out in the back and just gradually moving ahead of other runners. I did not use a heart rate monitor while racing as I am very familiar with how I feel when I run and what my heart rate is. I tried to pretty much run in a range of 130 to 150 bpm. I did have to cut back on weekly mileage to about 30 miles per week, and the mileage of each outing to less than one hour of running. I also cut back on the intensity or pace of my runs. The biggest thing I noticed was my breathing was more labored especially as I got bigger and I had to be more concerned about my balance. I also needed to take a few more days off then usual as in general I was more tired.*
>
> *During my second pregnancy I was not able to run much at all after the first trimester. My second child carried much lower in my pelvis and it was painful to run. I was able to maintain my fitness level by swimming, using the elliptical machine, and occasionally running in the pool.*
>
> *I was extremely nauseous well into the second trimester during both pregnancies. This only occasionally interfered with running, but I had to be very careful to stay hydrated. Physically I felt great."*

While Sue doesn't think that her fitness influenced her delivery (she had both children by C-section as her first child was upside down in the birth canal), she believes that being an athlete helped her to a speedy recovery. She ran the first leg (3 miles) of a marathon relay about 3 weeks after her second child was born!

Running In Later Pregnancy

"I felt the strongest, lots of energy ... no morning sickness," recalls a world class runner about the second trimester of her pregnancy. Yes, it's true, at midpoint (four to seven months) you may feel your best, but you'll also be aware of the added weight and minor aches and pains. It is time to slow down, decrease your mileage, and consider some running alternatives.

Most women I interviewed cut back their mileage 30 to 40 per cent by the second trimester and up to 70 per cent in the last weeks. Some women stopped running altogether because of the extra weight and abdominal pressure. Your running gait changes so be alert to terrain and traffic. You tend to not pick your feet up as high and your stride shortens.

I used to daydream while running. I would think about the growing being inside me or sort through baby names in my mind until loose pavement or an oncoming car would get me back in focus. I learned to stay alert and run cautiously.

If running becomes uncomfortable, consider non-weight bearing options for exercise. As a runner, you've probably already engaged in cross-training activities. If you are planning a pregnancy and run exclusively, now, before conception, is the time to introduce yourself to some other activities. In other parts of this book, you can review such options as swimming, paddling, cycling, cross country skiing, Nordic track, low impact aerobics, and walking. Find an activity or two that you can safely enjoy throughout your pregnancy.

> "I was running 50 miles per week before I was pregnant, and actually felt good and fast running for the first trimester. I tapered down to 35 miles per week (also slower pace) by 5 months, and then stopped completely. I very suddenly just started feeling very tired trying to run. My exercise from months 5 to 7 was mostly ice skating and downhill skiing and walking. For the last 2 months I have been walking. I'm most comfortable doing 3-4 short walks per day totaling 4-6 miles."
> Mother of four

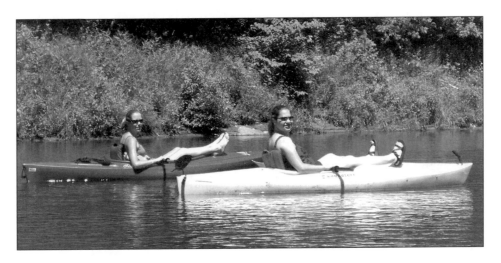

If running becomes uncomfortable, consider non-jarring options.

Jessica started running when she was 10 years old. She ran cross country and outdoor track through middle school, high school, and into college. She continues to compete in many local road races. Jessica discusses running, racing, and running/racing with a baby jogger.

"I conceived mid-November and I continued to run normally for a while, but with winter weather and experiencing fatigue from the first trimester, I took it easy. I participated in a local 5K race at 6 weeks, in which I monitored my heart rate, and I placed in my age group. After that I continued to run, but went easy to keep my heart rate low. After 4-5 months, I felt a bit uncomfortable so I started just doing a walking routine. Within in a couple weeks, I started becoming very grumpy, as my body really missed the endorphins. So I started running again and stopped around 7 months. I then committed myself to a walking routine. I continued my walking routine, walking 3 or more miles. The day I went into labor, I had walked 3.5 miles that morning.

I was hoping that my athleticism would influence my childbirth experience. It did not. The pain of labor is much different than enduring a marathon. I do think that being an athlete contributed to an easy pregnancy.

My daughter loves riding in the baby jogger. Her longest run is about 14 miles. She does 3-4 miles with me often. I just load up the baby jogger with something to drink and snack on. I did a 10K race with her when she was 9 weeks old. She has done a couple other races, and would do more, but many races now exclude baby joggers. I still run, but have not signed up for a marathon, wanting to spend my time with family instead."

Walking

Walking is a good, safe alternative throughout your pregnancy. It is less jarring and puts less stress on your ligaments and joints. If done using correct form and with purpose, walking can be just as invigorating as running and a welcome change.

Sore ligaments, pelvic pressure, Braxton Hicks contractions and urinary frequency are common "end stage" complaints and force many women to cut back or cease running. Substituting walking for running or alternating running and walking is a great way to move through the later part of pregnancy. Unless a medical problem intervenes, make your own decision as to when to cutback or stop your running.

One of the great things about walking is that you and your partner can share this activity, as well as some conversation, without the stress of trying to keep up with each other. Later, while pushing a baby stroller you will be "strolling," but now, during your pregnancy, you will most likely be walking at a brisk 14 to 18 minute per mile pace.

Walking Tips

- Shoes. You may want to buy a shoe specifically designed for walking if you plan to walk a lot. A walking shoe has a lower heel (1/2 inch) versus a running shoe which is usually 3/4 inch. A lower, more firm heel is less tiring for walking.
- Walking gait. Like your running gait, your walking gait is also altered in the later months of your pregnancy. When walking briskly, you need to pay attention to your posture and arm and leg swing. Keep your head straight with your chin parallel to the ground. Avoid looking down. Like running, you want to keep your head up and look forward. Your shoulders need to be loose and level. Try to keep your hips under your shoulders avoiding a sway back. Your stride length should be what normally feels comfortable.
- Arm swing. Just like in running, your arms play an important role in helping you move faster and more efficiently. The arms counterbalance and complement your legs as you move. Bend your arm at the elbow so it forms a 90 degree angle. Keep your elbow locked as you swing it toward the front stopping as the hand just reaches the center of your chest. Swing it back until it reaches just about mid-buttocks. Put some force and power in your arm swing. Forget arm and leg weights — they alter your normal arm and leg swing and may cause injury. Besides, you're carrying enough added weight.

Hiking

Hiking is a pleasurable activity you can enjoy throughout your pregnancy. Day hikes with your partner or friends provide an opportunity to explore nature while getting some exercise. Hiking is also an activity you can continue later on with your baby in a carrier or with young children for short outings.

As with any sport or activity, you need to dress for the weather, especially if you will be changing elevation. Layer your clothing or carry extra gear in a backpack along with snacks and water. Lightweight hiking shoes are comfortable and durable. You need a higher boot for added support if you are hiking any distance or over changing terrain. Remember, your joints and ligaments (especially your ankles in this case) are vulnerable to strains or sprains. Wear a comfortable pair of socks with extra padding to prevent friction and blisters.

Use common sense. Avoid rugged terrain, "bushwhacking," steep ascents or slick conditions. Stick with familiar trails or ones you have mapped out carefully. County, state, or national parks often have well-marked trails as well as

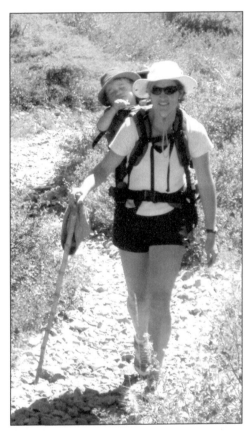

Hiking is a great activity to continue with your baby or young children for short outings.

bathroom facilities. You should not hike at altitudes over 8,000 feet due to the decrease in oxygen at higher elevations. Regardless of the altitude, keep a safe comfortable pace with frequent rest and water stops. The fresh air, the solitude, and the slower pace provide an opportunity to move with your thoughts while getting some exercise.

"Swimming helped me prepare for the intensity of labor. It helped me to cope with the physical demands of labor much better." A mother who swam during pregnancy

Chapter 10

Swimming and Water Activities

Swimming

I spent some of my most pleasurable memories during pregnancy submerged in water staring at a blue line at the bottom of a swimming pool. My view rolled with each stroke, one moment the lit pool room and the next moment the blue line below as I rhythmically breathed with each stroke. The water buoyed my expanding abdomen — I felt less big — less awkward — less pregnant! No doubt about it, swimming felt great!

I usually swam in the morning which helped lessen my bouts with nausea and gave me more energy for working during the day. In the water, my mind would wander to thoughts of the baby inside — imagining what he or she might be feeling as we rhythmically moved through the water. The baby tended to be less active during these early morning workouts. "Probably napping," I thought.

If you swam as a fitness activity before you became pregnant, there's an excellent chance you will be able to continue from conception right up to the delivery of your baby. "I stopped the day before my baby was born," reported an experienced swimmer who swam throughout her pregnancy. Another, who did the same, said, "I finished swimming one hour before my labor began. During early labor you may even find yourself submerged in water in a tub at your hospital or birthing center. Warm water is a great muscle relaxer and pain reliever.

If you are planning pregnancy in the future, now would be a good

You are less likely to overheat while swimming because the water surrounding your body keeps you cool while exercising. The rhythmic breathing in swimming is great practice for relaxed breathing during your labor. Try visualizing your labor while doing laps and maintaining a rhythmic pattern of slow, deep breathing. Stay relaxed and focused.

time to brush up on your swimming technique. Swimming may end up being the one exercise that will get you through the last lap of pregnancy. If you are a scuba diver, retire your wet suit and tank during pregnancy — the risks to the fetus in a submerged environment are not known at this point.

As mentioned previously, the hormones of pregnancy relax your joints and ligaments making them vulnerable to injury. The buoyancy of water provides you with a gentle buffer against strain and injury. Swimming helps you build endurance and strengthen and tone your muscles, especially your arms and legs. When you are submerged in water, fluid in your tissues is forced back into your bloodstream. This process helps reduce swelling, a common problem later in pregnancy. Pregnant swimmers notice more of an urge to empty their bladders. This is the way your body gets rid of the extra fluid so be sure to empty your bladder right before a swim and be prepared to take a bathroom break.

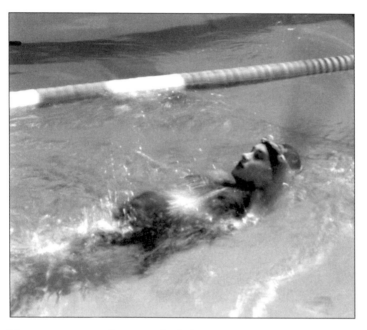

The water surrounding your body keeps you cool while exercising.

"I found I craved that time in the water because it was a way to get exercise and be off my feet. It gave me a full-body work out." Gayle, former college swimmer

Into The Pool

Before continuing your swim program, discuss your plans with your health care provider. Let him or her know how often and how long you are swimming, at what intensity, and how you are feeling as your pregnancy progresses. Remember, you are swimming to maintain your fitness, not to train or compete. This is the time to really tune into your body and listen to any signals it might be sending.

► *What To Wear?*

Maternity swimsuits create more drag because of the extra material that acts as a "cover up." You will probably be more comfortable in a nylon or Lycra® one piece suit, a size or two larger. Besides, why "hide" your pregnancy? A sports bra worn underneath will help give extra support and reduce breast tenderness. "I wore my old stretched out suits, some 'junk' suits from a friend and bought one suit in a bigger size," one swimmer told me. A swim cap keeps your hair out of your eyes and helps protect your hair against the damage of chlorine. Special shampoos to eliminate chlorine are a good idea. Goggles protect your eyes from irritation and improve your vision.

► *Ready — Set — Go!*

The temperature of the pool should be between 83 and 86 degrees. Warmer temperatures may cause overheating and cooler temperatures will cause excessive heat loss and shivering. Schedule your swim when the pool is least crowded. Sharing a lane with a "lane hog" can be frustrating and potentially dangerous. You also end up focusing more attention on the other swimmer which takes away the enjoyment of your swim.

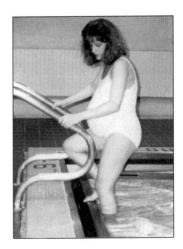

Use the ladder to enter and exit the pool.

Before getting into the pool, empty your bladder and do a few stretches for your arms and legs. Avoid jumping into the pool feet first due to the rare possibility of water being forced into your vagina. For safety's sake, don't dive after the first trimester. Start off slowly and gradually pick up your pace after you are warmed up. Always swim in a supervised pool or if you are swimming in a lake, with a buddy.

Most of you can continue to do all swim strokes — freestyle (crawl), backstroke, and breaststroke — that you normally use for workouts. More experienced swimmers can still do the butterfly — which requires more energy and technique. Whatever stroke you use, concentrate on good form and stroke technique to move your changing body efficiently through the water. Keep your strokes long and relaxed. Try to get as much distance as possible with each stroke. Just as in other sports, it's safest to eliminate speedwork and competition unless you are an elite swimmer under the guidance of a health care professional.

► Freestyle

For the freestyle stroke, your palms should be facing your feet with each stroke. Your hands, not your elbows, lead the pull of the stroke. Keep the waterline at your hairline. When breathing, allow your head to move independently of your upper body. Lift and turn your head with your neck. As soon as you take a quick breath, return to the face down position. The underwater arm pull in the freestyle is an elongated "S," keeping your elbow bent, up to 90 degrees. Your elbow is high while your forearm is completely relaxed. Your hand enters the water at a 45 degree angle in front of your shoulders.

In later pregnancy, your expanding abdomen will create more drag (resistance) in the water. The tendency will be for you to kick harder using up more energy. Keep your kicks small and moderate or consider wearing fins to give you more propulsion. Relax your ankles and bend your knees slightly on the downbeat, straightening them on the upbeat. Only your heels should be breaking the surface.

► Breaststroke

Relaxation in your hips and pelvis from the hormones of pregnancy make the frog kick of the uncomfortable. Try slowing down your kick and keep your knees closer together. Leslie, an experienced swimmer, as well as other swimmers I spoke with, felt soreness in their lower backs during the breastroke. Posture adjustments in pregnancy cause an increase in the curvature of your lower spine. The breastroke may exacerbate this problem.

► Backstroke

Some women I spoke with felt fine doing the backstroke in later pregnancy while others felt more awkward. The profile of your abdomen cruising through the water will certainly be an eye opener at your pool. If you feel uncomfortable backstroking, stick with the freestyle and breaststroke during your pregnancy.

> *"I felt less coordinated on my back. It was hard to keep good form with the added heaviness of my abdomen."* Karen at eight months

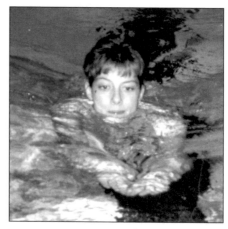

Breastroke

Choose the strokes that feel most comfortable for you and be willing to modify according to how you feel on any given day. What about flip turns? Most women eliminate these as they get bigger. One told me, "It was harder for me to get into a tuck for flip turns near the end of my pregnancy. It was more important for me to keep a steady pace during my swims." She also noted that she had to resort to using the ladder to get in and out of the pool — definitely "un-cool," in her words, since "real" swimmers make their exits out of the water on their arms.

► Training Devices

Training devices can add some fun and focus to your pool swims. Pull buoys, a flotation device placed between your legs, keeps your lower body buoyant while you concentrate on your arm stroke. Lisa, a triathlete, used a pull buoy to match the buoyancy of her growing abdomen. She found that her legs tended to sink without the pull buoy.

Hand paddles come in various sizes and help strengthen your shoulders, chest and back. The added resistance makes your upper bodywork harder. If you haven't used these before pregnancy, don't start now. They require good technique and might cause injury if not used properly.

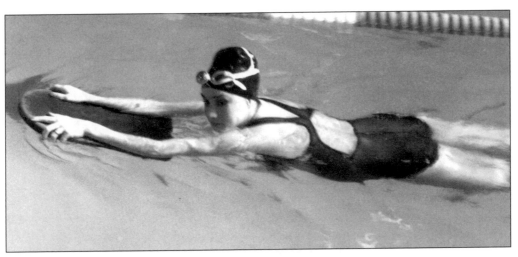

A kickboard can help you strengthen your lower body.

A kickboard allows you to build leg strength and concentrate on your kick. Kathy, a mother of three, used a kickboard for swimming during her second pregnancy. At the time, she was not a strong swimmer so she placed the board under her chest for added buoyancy and proceeded to do lap after lap, kicking all the way! You can use a kickboard to break up your swim and strengthen your lower body. A few swimmers I spoke with noticed a jump in their heart rates while kicking with a board. Your heart has to work harder to pump oxygen to your working leg muscles. Slow the kick down and rest longer between laps.

Swim fins help you develop ankle flexibility and stroke technique. The propulsion of the fins provides stability and balance. Fins can help you overcome the added drag of your growing abdomen and still maintain good form. It's a great feeling to cruise along as your feet flutter effortlessly. Try them and enjoy the ride!

Gayle got an early start to swimming, joining her town's summer league as a five year old. At eight years, she joined a swim team and competed all through high school. She attended the University of Denver on scholarship, swimming for three years, and now continues to swim on a regular basis. Gayle, mother of two boys, shares her pregnancy training routine.

"During my first pregnancy I swam 3 to 4 times a week for about an hour. I was working out with a small group at Johnson State College. I continued to swim intervals and train with the others for most of my pregnancy. I found that towards the very end stages (last month) of my pregnancy, I was more or less just swimming and not pushing myself as much. Although, I was surprised I was able to do flip turns through my whole pregnancy. I did not do butterfly in the last stages, but did continue to do the dolphin kick with a kickboard. I also found the backstroke made me lightheaded in the final month.

I did swim during my second pregnancy, but because I had a two year old at home I found I was only getting out about two times per week. I did do the swim leg of a triathlon at 35 weeks and was absolutely fine!

I loved being pregnant and felt great my first time around. I found I did not show early on and always got comments on how small I looked even later in my pregnancy. Swimming was amazing for me. I found I craved that time in the water because it was a way to get exercise and be off my feet. It gave me a full-body work out. I also think doing flip turns throughout the pregnancy was extremely beneficial. My stomach shrunk down within a few weeks and I was back into most of my pre-pregnancy clothes. I also found it did not take me long to recover. I was back hiking within three weeks of delivering.

I had two natural births. My second labor was very short. During both childbirths my final pushing stage was very short. My first one I pushed for 10 minutes and my second one I pushed two times! I spent both of my labors in the birthing tub and delivered my second son in the water. For me this was the only place I could let my body relax and stay focused. I feel my experience as an athlete gave me the necessary skills to focus and endure natural childbirth.

As a mother, I never put my two sons in a baby tub. They always went in the tub with me or in a sponge pad in the bathtub. My first son was 10 months and my second was four months when they first were introduced to a swimming pool. They both went under water by a year. We spend a lot of time in the water. Both sons were swimming briefly on their own by two and my oldest was completely on his own by the age of three. They are both very comfortable in the water."

Water Exercise

Water aerobics and water exercise, like swimming, use the buoyancy and resistance of water for a beneficial, non-weight bearing workout. The buoyancy of the water prevents jarring and jerky movements and puts less strain on your limbs and joints. At the same time, the resistance of the water helps you build strength, endurance and flexibility. It also may help avoid lower back pain: a study of 390 healthy pregnant women in Sweden showed a significant decrease in lower back pain with women who exercised using water aerobics once a week.

You can find water aerobics classes at many YWCA's, community pools, and health clubs. Check to see if there is a special prenatal water aerobics class in your area. Don't eat right before class and wear a comfortable suit with a supportive bra. If you wear glasses, stabilize them with a headband before getting in the water. Movements in the water are choreographed to music. (A boom box really bangs it out in a pool room — your baby will love it!) Use a full range of motion with slower, yet forceful movements for your arms and legs. Bigger movements push more water, giving you a better workout. Sometimes hand held devices like paddles or jugs are used

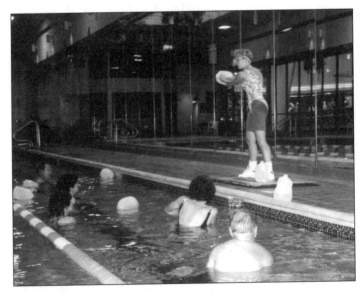

If you attend a regular water aerobics class, let the instructor know that you are pregnant and exercise at your own pace.

to create more resistance when working the arms and shoulder muscles. Keep your breathing even. Be aware of any signs of strain. Stop or modify the movement if you feel discomfort or pain. You should be able to carry on a conversation or sing along with the music during your workout. Keep your intensity level at 12 to 14 on the Rate of Perceived Exertion Scale (See Chapter 3).

Remember that even when you're in the water, you still perspire so you need to drink plenty of water before, during and after your workouts. Always keep a water bottle nearby and try to take a drink every 10 minutes or so.

A workout in the pool keeps your heart rate lower than the same workout on land. The physiological effects of being submerged in water is responsible for this "user-friendly" response. Exercising in water keeps you cooler and prevents overheating. However, you still need to drink plenty of water before and after your workout. Classes end with gentle stretching to bring your heart rate down and relax your muscles.

If a water aerobics class is not available where you live, you can use the pool for some water calisthenics or walking and jogging in place. Flotation belts or vests keep you vertical for walking or jogging. Design your own water workout — let those creative juices flow! Use a kickboard or hold on to the edge of the pool for legwork or kicking. Work both your lower and upper body. Keep the movements big and make sure your breathing is slow and relaxed. End your workout with some gentle stretching.

Paddling & Rowing

Being in the water feels terrific while you are pregnant, but so does being on the water. Paddling a canoe or kayak, or rowing in a shell are some non-impact aerobic activities that translate well into the physiological changes of pregnancy. The craft supports your weight so there is little risk of injury to your joints or ligaments from heavy impact. Paddling gets you outdoors where you can savor the peace and beauty of a lake or river.

When I lived near a lake, I was provided with many pleasurable early morning paddles on clear, calm waters. The simple task of thrusting a paddle into water and powering the movement of a sleek Kevlar canoe is my version of a great wake-up call. I tried to get out shortly after sunrise when sometimes I would meet a lone fishing boat or a covey of ducks on the journey up the west side of the lake. I gazed ahead at the bow of the canoe and watch the water being displaced by the power of my efforts. By the turn-around, the wind had picked up, and now, with the wind at my back, I headed home. I struggled to stay flat and keep a straight course. Once at the shoreline, I paused, and sitting in the canoe, gazed at the still-quiet lake. I paddled right up to delivery, always enjoying a refreshing morning workout.

Paddling a canoe or a kayak is a sport open to women of all ages and athletic backgrounds, from the recreational paddler to the serious competitor. Women are well suited for paddling; most of the power comes from your back and torso.

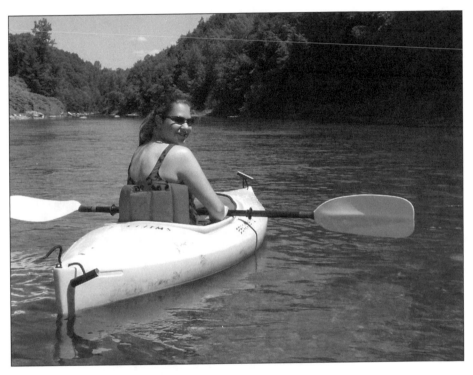

Stick with a stable boat and calm waters.

For recreational purposes, a standard canoe made of aluminum or fiberglass fits the bill. Serious competitors move up to sleek racing canoes. Likewise, kayaks come in many varieties but you'll want to use a very stable one with plenty of cockpit space. Drinking systems consist of jugs and tubing for "no hands" drinking but you can just carry a couple of water bottles. Replenishing fluids is important for distance racing.

Rowing began as an intercollegiate sport for women in the sixties and seventies. It became an Olympic sport for women in 1976. Since then, women at all levels, high school, college, clubs, and masters participate in crew. Shells come in one, two, four, or eight person models. Sculling is rowing with two oars per oarswoman. Sweep rowing is rowing with one oar per person on the right or left side of the shell. Events are classified as heavyweight (shells with a rower weighing more than 130 pounds) or lightweight (all rowers weight less than 130 pounds). The rower slides fore and aft on the seat with each stroke. When you place the oar in the water (catch phase), flex your knees, hips and back and extend your elbows. Your legs, as well as your arms, chest, and back help to power the shell during the propulsion phase when the oar(s) pulls you through the water. Watching a shell moving through the water makes you appreciate the rhythm and pulse of this water sport.

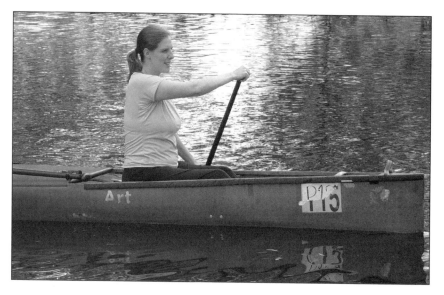

Keep your strokes easy and just enjoy being on the water.

Paddling Or Rowing During Pregnancy

Whether you paddle or row competitively or recreationally, you can safely continue either of these activities by making some minor adjustments and modifications during your pregnancy. Now is the time to tame your adventurous spirit and stick with calm waters on a familiar lake or flat river. Avoid strong currents, fast water or heavy boat traffic. In windy conditions, it's best to stay closer to shore to lessen the effects. Always paddle or row with a partner. Carry a PFD (personal flotation device) or wear it if you are not a strong swimmer. Dress for comfort and ease of movement. A T-shirt over cycling shorts or shorts with an adjustable waist band works well. Protect yourself from the sun with sunblock, a hat and sunglasses. Water sport shoes or light running shoes are fine. For cooler weather dress in layers and wear light gloves.

Susan, an experienced marathon canoe racer, paddled throughout her first pregnancy. In her first trimester she did shorter races at a comfortable pace and stayed well hydrated. For Susan, paddling felt very comfortable, more so than running where she experienced Braxton Hicks contractions in the last trimester. She attributes her triumph, Stella (eight pounds), delivered after a 21 hour labor, to her physical fitness and mental toughness.

Be prepared to make some adjustments. You may need to adjust the seats as your weight changes over the next nine months to keep the boat moving level. Getting in and out of one of a "squirrelly" canoe or kayak can be tricky at eight or nine months. Use a stable craft and take it slowly. Your stroke will change due to the bulk of the baby, especially in the sitting position. You will not be able to rotate your torso as much and may need to shorten your stroke a bit. Keep the strokes steady and easy. Avoid speedwork or sprints, just enjoy being on the water.

Rowing, also a non-weight bearing activity, is a great sport to continue during your pregnancy, either indoors on a rowing ergometer, or on the water in a shell. Rowing, unlike paddling, involves both upper and lower body movements. Sculling or sweeping involves flexion of your knees, back and elbows. Practice good technique and modify if necessary to avoid injury to your relaxed joints and ligaments. For instance, you'll need to shorten your stroke in later pregnancy due to the "second passenger." You may need to reduce the load of rowing by shortening your oars or increasing the inboard length or flex of the oars, although doing this may cause the oar to land closer to your abdomen. Rowing on an ergometer has the added advantage of keeping you cool from the back draft of the flywheel. Put on a pair of headphones for entertainment. Keep a water bottle at your side and stay at a comfortable pace.

"I always listened to my respiratory rate and how I actually felt. I am a true believer in knowing your own body and listening to that. You have to be honest with yourself." A former nationally-ranked competitive cyclist and mother of three

Chapter 11

Cycling

Riding a bike is not only fun but has health benefits too. Since cycling is a non-weight bearing activity, it spares your joints and ligaments while providing many benefits. Your heart and lungs become more efficient at pumping oxygen to the working muscles in your legs. If you use pedal straps or a cleated shoe, your legs become stronger as they pull the pedals around each stroke. Your upper body is basically in a static position, nevertheless your back, arms, and abdomen are all working to hold you upright as your legs do the work of pedaling. Cycling, especially when combined with other activities like running or swimming, is a great way to stay healthy and fit.

Cycling has mental benefits also. The women cyclists I spoke with convinced me that "runner's high" has its biological equivalent in cycling. The feelings of elation, contentment and confidence are common for dedicated cyclists. Cycling outdoors rewards you with the sights and sounds along your journey and the chance to clear your head. Whether you ride a mountain bike or road bike, you will be greeted by a sense of freedom and adventure on the ride.

Before we talk about cycling in pregnancy, I want to discuss cycling in general: types of bikes, proper fit, equipment and clothing, and safety issues. A discussion of these points will help you make a safe transition from cycling solo to cycling for two.

Types Of Bikes

As the interest in cycling has grown, so has the industry of bike designs. The bikes we learned on seem obsolete, replaced by a variety of models that fit each person's lifestyle and fitness goals.

► *Sport Touring Bike*
Once the most popular type of bike (before the advent of mountain bikes), a sport bike still provides an economical entry into cycling. It usually has ten or twelve speeds

and is suitable for either recreational or fitness riding. Given their stability, ease-of-riding, they are perfectly-suited for riding during pregnancy.

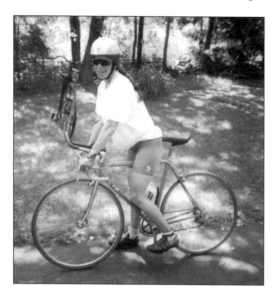

Returning from a ride on a sport/racing bike.

► *Loaded Touring Bikes*

If you have a travel bug, this is the bike that will get you there and back. These bikes are designed to carry panniers (large bike bags) or bike racks. Touring bikes have a longer wheel base (the distance between the center of the front axle and rear axle) which makes the ride smoother. A third chainring adds extra low gearing for climbing hills. You need this low gearing when you're riding with twenty or thirty pounds of gear.

► *Racing Bikes*

Racers want to go fast, and these bikes are designed to do just that. The gearing is narrower, which means that it is geared higher for speed. The high pressure, narrow tires meet less resistance on the pavement. "Aero" bars are popular with triathletes and time trialists. They reduce wind resistance by keeping you riding low.

► *Mountain Bikes*

Whether you ride on trails or roads, these versatile bikes are very popular and easy to ride. Equipped with fat tires, upright handlebars and a triple chainring for wide range gearing, mountain bikes are designed for rugged terrain — whether it's climbing a rocky pass or descending a mountain trail. They also are great around town if you like to sit upright and ride on wide stable tires. If you mountain bike while pregnant, stay off the trails and stick to back roads and bike paths.

► *Hybrid Bikes*

Hybrids are a cross between a mountain and road bike. They are sturdy enough to handle more rugged terrain and yet they can cruise along the road at a good pace. You can get performance wheels for them, which are perfect for road riding, or slightly fatter wheels and tires for more rugged conditions. Their flat handlebars allow a more upright riding position. They are the favorite of bike touring companies due to their versatility – and they may become your favorite as well. Given their stability and upright ride, they are a good option for cycling while pregnant.

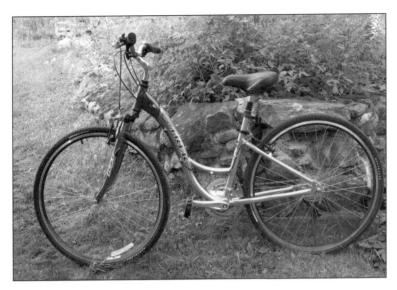

A hybrid may be a good option during pregnancy.

Correct Fit

No matter what type of bike you're riding, correct fit is essential. If you're not comfortable, you're not having fun. Incorrect fit can lead to injury and frustration. The first bike I bought did not fit properly. The salesperson had me straddle the top tube to measure the clearance between the crotch and tube (one to two inches) — and that was it. I never felt comfortable on the bike. Before buying my next bike, I did some research.

Most bikes are designed around male anatomy. Our bodies have some significant differences which need to be considered when fitting a bike. We tend to have shorter arms and torso, longer legs, narrower shoulders, a wider pelvis and smaller hands. Many bikes, designed for men, tend to feel to stretched out for us. So, how do you get a bike that fits correctly and handles well?

More and more major manufacturers are offering woman-sized bicycles. These stock bikes usually have shorter stems and top tubes as well as a woman's saddle. However, if they use standard-size wheels (700c), there may be compromises in frame angles that can result in a less than optimum pedaling position for you. But check it out – particularly ones that use smaller (650c) wheels.

Another option is to "retrofit" a bike. A Fit Kit is a fitting aid which can help you do this by making adjustments to fit your proportions. A common practice for women is to replace the handlebar stem with a shorter one. This brings the handlebars closer to the seat to accommodate our shorter arms and torso. Call your local bike shop to see if this is available. I used a Fit Kit when I bought my second bike. I bought a frame and then built the bike around my proportions.

What about a bike designed for women by women? Terry Precision road bikes have been leaders in designing bicycles for women's frames and offer a wide range of stock bicycles and cycling gear.

Another option is a custom bike. Custom bicycles cost more – each one is built individually and the materials are often lighter and better, and more expensive. Talk to your bike shop staff for ideas and work with a designer who is familiar with women's anatomy. You may find that if you have to make expensive modifications to get a stock bike fitting you, that a custom purchase may not be that much more. (See the Resource Section for several builders.)

Besides proper frame size and fit, you need to consider a few other things to ensure a comfortable ride.

Saddles

It's important to ride on a saddle that fits you and your riding style. Your pelvis is wider than a man's. The bones you sit on (ischial tuberosities) are further apart and may need a slightly wider seat. Many saddle manufacturers make "women's" models which are a little shorter and anywhere from a little to a lot wider than regular saddles. You can buy "anatomic" seats which are slightly wider and shorter and have extra padding for the ischial. Some of them have cut-outs or perforations in the saddle shell which, along with the shorter nose, help alleviate some of the pressure of the contact points. Terry Precision, the fore-mentioned women-owned company, makes a line of saddles which are popular with many women riders. Check out the saddles and find one that is comfortable.

A common error novice riders make is to ride with the seat too low or too high. Remember, whenever you adjust the saddle height, you are altering the action of every muscle involved in pedaling. Set your seat height by sitting, without shoes, on the seat, placing the pedal at the bottom of the stroke. Your knee should be slightly bent. (It helps to have your partner or a bike shop technician do this with you.) Your saddle should be level to distribute your weight evenly.

Pedals

Efficient pedaling requires that your feet be properly placed on the pedals. The strapless pedal binding system is a great improvement over the toe clip and allows you to fine tune the placement of your feet. You can prevent injuries, like knee pain, by fine tuning the angle of your cleats. A Fit Kit can help you properly align the cleats on the shoe. To release your foot, you just rotate your heel outward. The toe clip requires that you reach down and release the strap. Many shoes are compatible with the newer binding systems. It's a good idea to put away the clipless pedals during pregnancy and stick to either loose toe clips or straight pedals.

Equipment And Clothing

Never ride without a helmet. Whether you have a mountain or road bike, you need to protect your head. Over 75% of cycling deaths result from head injuries. You're also setting an example for younger riders. Fortunately, most states have established laws that mandate helmets for children. Make sure your helmet has a certification sticker — older helmets should have ANSI, Snell, or ASTM stickers: new ones should meet the CPSC uniform safety standard.

If you do much cycling, flat tires are inevitable. You're cruising along, enjoying the ride, and the next thing you know, you are sitting beside the road, fixing a flat tire. Always carry a spare tube, tire levers, and pump. CO_2 cartridges are handy for fast inflations. Practice a tire change at home beforehand.

Sunglasses protect you from ultraviolet rays but they also keep flying objects — like bugs — out of your eyes. The wrap around style usually works best. Again, glasses are usually designed for men so try to get a narrower frame that fits comfortably.

Drink before you go and always carry water on your rides. Dehydration can be dangerous, especially in hot and humid conditions. You need to drink at least 16 ounces of water for every hour of cycling. Avoid the sports drinks. Replacement drinks contain ingredients that are not necessary for moderate levels of exercise and their use in pregnancy has not been studied. They also may upset your stomach. One competitive cyclist, who usually drank sports drinks while training, told me that she was unable to tolerate this during her early pregnancy. She said, "It made me even more nauseated while riding."

Cycling clothing is comfortable and aerodynamic. Non-restrictive shorts and jerseys made of a lycra/spandex material are the most popular because they increase your comfort by wicking away sweat from your body. Buy shorts designed for women which avoid center seams and are usually lined with a cotton blend or fleece fabric. The back pockets on a cycling jersey are handy for carrying quick snacks, identification, a lightweight jacket, or keys. (The pockets are located on the back instead of the sides to prevent them from rubbing against your legs while you pedal.) Besides lycra, jerseys are available in a variety of fabrics with less "cling." Cotton T-shirts work fine with a supportive bra. Some women like the baggy shorts with a crotch lining for mountain biking or touring. Bright colors and reflective piping are good safety features.

In cooler weather, some of us head indoors (see Indoor Cycling) while the rest of us just add layers. You can wear a pair of Lycra® tights over your cycling shorts and then peel them off once you've warmed up. There are a variety of fabrics and designs for jackets and tights which wick away moisture to keep you warmer. Shoe covers keep your feet warm.

Cycling gloves prevent blister and "road rash" — the painful outcome when skin meets pavement. A gloved hand can also brush off debris from your tires. The fingerless style is great for warmer weather but you will want a full glove with a good grip in cooler temperatures.

Safety

Sharing the road is the credo of cycling. But remember, you're sharing it with big heavy objects! Stay alert and ride defensively. Here are some general safety tips.

- Obey all traffic rules. This sounds simple but there are times when it's tempting to blow through a stop light or signal. This attitude not only doesn't help relations with motorists — it is also dangerous.
- Stay to the right except in turn lanes when you want to give way to turning vehicles.
- Ride single file and stay as close to the shoulder as possible.
- Signal your intentions with hand signals.

- Watch for road hazards like potholes, rocks, gratings, and railroad tracks. A triathlete friend had the misfortune of being thrown from her bike while crossing railroad tracks during a race. She suffered a fractured clavicle. Always approach tracks head on and not at an angle.
- Stay alert. Leave your headphones at home.
- Deal smartly with dogs. A blast with your water bottle or a verbal counter attack — (GET BACK!!) may ward off the barking beast. Small blast horns are available that fit in the palm of your hand and send off a piercing "stop dead in your tracks" noise. You can always dismount and place your bike between you and the dog.
- Ride with a partner when possible. Avoid isolated roads or trails or riding in the dark.
- Always let someone know your cycling route. Carry identification and spare change.
- Keep your bike tuned up and ready for the road or trails.

Two On The Bike

Cycling during your pregnancy is a great way to stay in shape. As mentioned earlier, because it is a non-weight bearing activity, you reduce the risk of injury to your relaxed joints or ligaments. As your pregnancy progresses, your changing center of gravity and increasing weight may make cycling a better option than running or cross country skiing. Perhaps cycling is already a part of your fitness program or an activity you pursued while nursing a running injury. Whether you have a road or mountain bike, or even a tandem, you can continue to cycle with modifications and adjustments. Be sure to check with your health care provider about your cycling program.

Your fitness goals for cycling will change during pregnancy. You are now riding to maintain fitness, not to train for competition. This can be a difficult transition if you are a competitive cyclist. A few experienced cyclists I spoke with said that they "participated" in citizen's races during the first few months of pregnancy. They cycled at a moderate pace (they were not racing) and stayed well hydrated. They were cycling for fun and fitness.

Cycling In Early Pregnancy

During the first few months of pregnancy, nausea and fatigue may cut your desire to exercise. Cycling may not sound appealing, but walking or swimming might be a good alternative. Some cyclists felt better getting outdoors in the fresh air. One competitive cyclist told me that she lost some of her ambition to ride in the early months due to fatigue. She rode less, cut back her mileage and felt better by the fourth month. Listen to your body in these first few months. Don't push it and be flexible.

Kathy, a cyclist for fourteen years and competitor for the last six years, felt a mixture of feelings early in her pregnancy. She was thrilled to be pregnant but also felt jealous of her former training partners as they cruised by her on their bikes early in her pregnancy. It helped for her to realize that her condition was temporary and the health of her baby was far more important. She continued to ride during her pregnancy, stopped all "training" and enjoyed riding for pleasure and fitness.

Urinary frequency and breast tenderness are common symptoms during pregnancy. Empty your bladder before a ride and try to plan a route where you can get to a bathroom or "outdoor facility." You might want to wear a small mini-pad just in case. Don't cut back on fluid replacement. Your body needs this to prevent dehydration and overheating. On the same note, avoid cycling in very hot or humid conditions.

A supportive bra or sports bra will help with tender breasts. A lycra top may feel too restrictive and uncomfortable so try a cotton T-shirt or loose fitting top.

Always stretch before getting on your bike (see Chapter 5). Focus on your hamstrings, calf muscles, Achilles tendons, hip flexors, neck and shoulders, and lower back. Start your ride spinning in easy gears. Likewise, at the end of the ride, shift to a cool down pace and replenish fluids. After long rides, be sure to eat some carbohydrates shortly after your cool down.

Cycling In Later Pregnancy

Your increasing weight and expanding abdomen, when coupled with your fetus's activity and position, may make cycling uncomfortable during the last few months of pregnancy. Many cyclists I interviewed had to alter their riding positions at this stage. Instead of riding on the drops (the lower portion of the drop handlebars), they rode in a more upright position with their hands on top of the handlebars. This gives more clearance for your abdomen, more room for lung expansion and puts less pressure on your hands. Some women switched to a mountain bike for the same reason.

When you ride on the drops, your hands and arms bear a good portion of your weight. Pressure on your hands, combined with the normal soft tissue swelling in pregnancy, can lead to nerve compression problems. The symptoms are numbness or tingling of the fingers, usually more painful at night. Let your health provider know if this is happening. Treatment is usually a wrist splint and ice packs.

Making some minor adjustments on your bike will make your ride more comfortable. Try moving your seat slightly forward to reduce the reach to the handlebars. Realize that by doing this, you are changing your pedaling form. You can also raise the handlebar stem gradually, a little each week. Keep the adjustments small. If you normally ride with aero bars, you may need to replace them with a traditional handlebar set for stability. When I found out that I was pregnant, one of the first things I did was retire my aero bars.

Some pregnant cyclists find that bib shorts and a t-shirt, supplemented with a supportive sports bra, makes a good outfit.

If you suffer from hemorrhoids, sitting in the saddle can be uncomfortable. Try one of the anatomic seats or a wider seat with extra padding. Lower backache is common in the last trimester. Strong abdominals as well as good posture and body mechanics will help prevent this problem. If back pain develops while riding, try different positions and maybe shorten your rides. Be sure to stretch your back before and after riding.

Braxton Hicks contractions, rhythmic tightenings of the lower abdomen, are common in the last trimester. Some cyclists experience these while riding, especially on longer rides. When these occur, slow down and focus on taking deeper breaths. If you're cycling on the drops, you are squeezing your diaphragm by both your position and your growing uterus. Your breathing becomes shallower. Try riding in the upright position or get off your bike, take a short rest, and drink some water.

Cycling may aggravate varicose veins. Because you are in a sitting position, you are further restricting blood flow to your legs. Support hose or lycra tights will provide some support. You will need to shorten your rides or switch to another exercise if they are severe or worsen with riding. Varicose veins in the vulvar area may be too uncomfortable for cycling altogether.

Vaginal yeast infections are common in pregnancy because of the rise in pregnancy hormones. Cycling can really irritate the situation because of the warm moist environment of cycling shorts and the friction of the bike seat. Change your shorts immediately after a ride. Try to wear shorts with the most breathable crotch lining.

Select fabrics which wick away moisture and are comfortable. Consult with your health care provider if this becomes a persistent problem.

Jan began racing in college and then competed on the US National Cycling Team. Her many cycling accomplishments include World Champion in 50K Women's Team Time Trial, Benidorm, Spain (1992); Silver Medal in 50K Women's Team Time Trial, Oslo, Norway (1993); and US National Cyclocross Champion (1995). Mother of three children, Jan says that each pregnancy was a little different in terms of riding.

"With my first child, I rode three to five days a week until the week before I delivered. I commuted twelve miles each way to work and would even fit in thirty minutes of lap swimming half way on the ride to the shop. I felt great. As I was in the last trimester during June, July, August, I slowed my speeds down to keep my body from getting very hot.

With my second child, I rode three days a week, mainly because of lack of time. Riding would be anywhere from a spin with Lucy in a child seat, to a two hour ride at a steady pace. I did a photo shoot with Bicycling Magazine two weeks before delivery and that was my last ride. Because of the way the baby sat inside, I was a little more uncomfortable in the bent over position.

With my third child, I was determined to still ride...time was certainly the issue. I felt great riding in the first two trimesters, as this was a winter baby (delivery 1/25/03), so I took to shoveling and sledding once I got to the winter months. At five months, my husband, Doug, and I rode many of the Alp passes for the 2002 Tour de France.

The first trimesters had their moments of the salivating mouth, but it was all bearable. Almonds would help to calm my stomach and hunger. I can remember feeling achy like I had the flu, but as soon as I would get going, I would feel better. Idle time was not good because that is when I would feel fatigued and tired. Exercise helped me during pregnancies to help me feel better about myself. It also helped me to stay with good eating habits. Exercise is ALWAYS a good thing for me mentally...it is my time, and I love to get out and breath and feel the outside air. The riding and other exercise helped me to have a strong and fit body throughout all the pregnancies.

With all three pregnancies, I was fortunate enough to not really begin to pop until the sixth month and my position on the bike did not change at all for at least the first five months.

I rode my regular road bike, which had a minimal 2-inch drop from seat to handlebars. Some days I felt as though I would try to support myself by pushing my upper body up from the handlebars. As the pregnancy continued, I had a very comfortable set up on a bike we set up as a commuter bike. The position had a 20-30 degree-rise stem, of shorter length. It was a flat handlebar with mountain bike levers. *The gearing was the same as road gearing, and the bike had narrow tires, like a traditional road bike. It was comfortable and nice to ride...I still ride it with the kids.*

I raced during pregnancies two and three. That was because I was not aware of being pregnant. I was in the third month with each of them and it was only one race. Once I learned I was pregnant, I did not race. With pregnancy one, I wore my heart rate monitor all of the time, but not with two and three. Even while wearing it during one, I always listened to my respiratory rate and how I actually felt. I am a true believer in knowing your own body and listening to that. You have to be honest with yourself. I stopped riding with others so I would not be tempted to ride harder. The heat also had in impact on my heart rate, by making it higher, so I continued to pay attention to my breathing. I would say that all of the riding was done in an aerobic state....being able to talk while I rode....even if it was to myself and the baby.

I believe the mental toughness of being an athlete helped me through labors. I would get into a race type of focus and breathe. My labors were four to eight hours. The conditioning over the years helped me to be able to endure the time when my body was taken over by labor. However, I still believe labor was the most difficult of any event I ever did. With racing and training you have the control to back off whenever, but with labor you have no control as to how long a contraction will be. It was unbelievable! I loved it! They were all natural deliveries".

How Fast? How Far? How Long?

The answers to these questions are individual. It will certainly depend on the health of your pregnancy and your level of fitness. Your cycling ability changes from early pregnancy to the last few months. Your center of gravity starts changing at about four months which may cause some balance problems. Your added weight means that you have to work harder to cycle. When cycling for two, you need to listen to the messages your body is sending.

Certainly you will need to avoid any anaerobic workouts like sprinting or intense speedwork. It's safer to ride at a constant level of intensity. Keep your workout at about 60 per cent to 75 per cent of your maximal heart rate. (See Chapter 3.) That's a "somewhat hard" workout, between 12 and 14, on the Rate of Perceived Exertion scale. Do not cycle to the point of exhaustion. If you need to rest right after riding, then your workout was too intense.

The distance you ride will depend on again your level of fitness and other factors like terrain and weather. Avoid steep hills and rough terrain. Choose rides that have smooth road conditions and alternate route options, in case you want to shorten the ride. We don't know the effects of polluted air while exercising in pregnancy, but using common sense, try not to cycle during the worst periods. If it's hazy, hot, and humid, cycle early in the day or indoors on a wind trainer with air conditioning. Drink plenty of fluids, before, during, and after the ride.

Sandy, a mother of two teenage daughters, cross country skied as well as cycled and swam during both her pregnancies. Her first daughter was conceived while on a 2,500-mile bike trip through Europe and England. Despite some nausea and emotional ups and downs ("At one point I broke down crying when a truck came too close to me") she and her husband completed the trek without mishap. Sandy swam throughout her first pregnancy and then picked up recreational cross country skiing during her last trimester. She and her husband back country skied into state lands and parks. "On the very day that Amy was born, I had planned to ski with my husband and another couple. I had to call it off because I went into labor," Sandy said. The birth was uncomplicated and Amy arrived weighing seven pounds, one ounce.

It sounds hard to believe, but Sandy conceived the second time while on a bike trip in New England. (What is it with bikes?) This time she skied all winter during her second trimester and felt great. She said, "I don't recall having any problems. In fact I did a 5 mile citizens' race and felt fine. I never pushed it." Sandy's labor and delivery was rapid, about 5 hours, and uncomplicated. Katrina weighed eight pounds, four ounces. Sandy gained about twenty pounds with both pregnancies and was back to her pre-pregnancy weight by her six week check-up.

I continued to cycle up to the day before I delivered — but with lots of modification. My pace slowed, and I tried to avoid steep hills and longer rides. My husband and I usually cycled together. We would agree on a route and then start out. He would cruise ahead and as soon as he was out of sight, circle back to me. I was glad we were able to both enjoy riding, and I know that he felt better knowing I wasn't cycling alone — which brings us back to the subject of safety.

All the safety issues previously discussed apply when cycling in pregnancy. Follow the rules of the road and carry identification and spare change. Avoid riding alone. Cycle with someone who matches your pace or do the "loop back" routine. Carry snacks and drink plenty of water. Stretch before and after your ride. Try to concentrate on good cycling form while making comfort adjustments as necessary. Be flexible.

Listen to your body for any of the following warning signs:

- Shortness of breath, dizziness or chest pain.
- Signs of labor: Regular contractions or leaking of water from the vagina.
- Vaginal bleeding.
- Decreased fetal movement.
- Pain in the hips, back or pelvic area.

Indoor Cycling

If you live in a part of the country where you can't cycle year round, or if you feel safer off the road or trail, then indoor cycling is a good alternative. An indoor bike is available year round, and in the later months, some of you may feel safer on a stationary bike. Changes in your sense of balance or poor weather can make indoor cycling sound appealing.

If you've never ridden a stationary bike, your first thought may be "BORING." Well, it can be, but find some interesting diversions like listening to music, reading, watching television, or letting your mind drift. Your thoughts may wander to your growing baby as you make mental lists of baby equipment. Also, video programs are available that simulate a bike ride.

A resistance trainer uses the back wheel of your bike to drive a resistance element. On a wind load simulator, the back tire makes contact with a shaft that turns a "squirrel" cage. A quieter model uses a magnetic device which rubs against the back tire. You can adjust for different levels of resistance. Place a board under the front wheel to keep your bike level and to avoid strain to your lower back. Rollers are a bit more tricky and probably not a good idea during pregnancy. You balance your bike while riding on top of rollers. A magnetic resistance unit is often attached to create resistance. A cloth shield is a smart accessory which shields your bike from sweat. Always ride in a cool room with fans or air-conditioning.

Health clubs generally have an array of computerized cycles. These can challenge your boredom with a variety of programs. While you monitor your performance, you can compete in a road race, ride on different types of terrain, or spin along at a steady pace. Fit is a problem with computerized cycles. The same "fit rules" apply as we discussed earlier. Check your seat height and the tilt of the saddle. Use the toe straps if available. You can adjust the handlebars in some models.

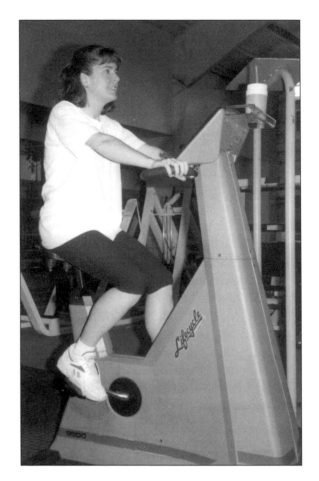

Indoor cycling machines have a variety of programs.

The Spinning® program is a way that some women make riding a stationary bike more fun. The great thing about Spinning is that it's a group format, but you ride your own ride. Basically, it's a mind/body workout, indoors on a stationary cycle that has a 39-pound fly wheel so it simulates the road. You control your own resistance with a knob on the bike. A certified instructor leads the class on a ride set to music. Rides are usually 40 minutes long, following safe guidelines like warm up, cool down and stretching. It is a good way to beat the boredom of indoor cycling.

Leah, Spinning® teacher and mother of two, scaled back her cycling program and integrated yoga as her pregnancies progressed:

> *"In my first trimester, I still rode outside, walked and taught three classes a week. I stopped riding technical trails in the woods, as I felt the risk of falling and taking a handle bar to the belly was far too great.*
>
> *As my pregnancy progressed and the seasons changed, outdoor riding was no longer part of my program. I found it difficult to teach, and get my own indoor rides in. So, I purchased a home Spinner and began to get my rides in the living*

room. *I also started prenatal yoga classes in my second trimester. I rode until my due date, and then found the bike just too uncomfortable. I was two weeks late, and in those last weeks, I walked often and practiced gentle yoga at home."*

Clothing

Early in pregnancy you can wear your regular cycling attire. A supportive bra or sports bra will help lessen irritation of tender breasts. In the heat you will want to wear breathable lightweight clothing. Cooler weather requires layering and fabric that wicks away moisture. In pregnancy, you tend to perspire more. Keep that in mind when dressing for cycling.

"I bought some padded maternity bike shorts, which were great and comfortable and a couple of maternity tanks that had a support bra insert. Dressing light was key." Cyclist and mother of two.

Later in pregnancy, your expanding abdomen will probably still fit inside your cycling shorts if you go up a size. Padded maternity bike shorts or bib cycling shorts are also options. (Some women like wearing a maternity belt for a more snug feel to the abdomen.) Traditional cycling jerseys may feel too restrictive, so try a large T-shirt that covers your abdomen. For safety, try to wear brightly colored clothes. Don't forget sunglasses, sunscreen, and your helmet.

"Skiing with a pulk has been the perfect way for my husband and I to get out skiing together and expose our daughter to our favorite winter activity, even if she's just riding. We had another baby this spring, so next winter will be more challenging but doable with a double pulk, toddler skiing (for 10 minutes), or taking turns in the lodge/skiing." Skier and mother of two

Chapter 12

Winter Activities

There is a popular 50-kilometer (31 miles) ski race in Central New York, called the Tug Hill Tourathon, which attracts cross country skiers of all levels from across the Northeast and Canada. This annual event takes place in one of the most beautiful and snow-laden regions in the state. Cold air moving across Lake Ontario creates "lake effect" snow — a snowmaking machine that dumps tons of snow over the whole area.

The first year I skied the race, a lake effect snowstorm made the car drive to the race treacherous. However, this didn't stop over 300 enthusiastic and determined skiers from lining up at the start. By then, the snow was coming down in large clumps, and the race directors told us that any tracks set earlier on the course were just a distant memory. As the gun went off, we plowed ahead through the ankle-deep fluffy snow.

Fortunately, the snow had tapered off by the 15 km mark, and skiers ahead had carved tracks for the rest of us. About then, I noticed a bobbing yellow sign up ahead hanging from the back of a skier. Approaching closer, I read the words, "BABY ON BOARD." As I moved to the outer tracks to pass, I noticed the protuberance at her waistline. "She must be in her seventh month," I thought.

The pregnant skier was moving along at a steady pace, rhythmically striding, looking comfortable, and obviously enjoying herself. Skiers around her offered words of encouragement and praise. Little did I know that the next time I skied the tourathon, I would be five months pregnant and skiing with my baby on board.

If you live where winter is snowy, the months from November to April can be a challenge. As we discussed in Chapter 9, the shorter days, icy conditions, and snowy roads can make running dangerous, especially during pregnancy. One alternative to running in slush, doing laps in the pool, or riding a wind trainer, is to strap on a pair of "skinny skis" and venture outdoors to cross country ski.

Cross country skiing is one of the best "total body" workouts. Unlike some other sports like running or cycling, skiing works both your upper and lower body — all your major muscle groups. It is a low impact sport with little risk of injury. Downhill skiing, on the other hand, probably should be discontinued during your later months of pregnancy. Your changing sense of balance can put you at risk for injury.

There are two basic techniques in cross country skiing. Classical skiing is the traditional method of skiing. Your arms and legs move in an exaggerated running motion as you glide across the snow in grooved tracks. Freestyle skiing, commonly called skating, is a technique of skating on skis where you transfer your weight from ski to ski as you glide on packed snow. Let's talk a bit about the technique and equipment in cross country skiing and then we'll discuss skiing in pregnancy.

Nordic Skiing For The Novice

If you have never cross country skied, now, during your pregnancy, is not the time to begin (you might, however, skip to the snowshoeing section further on). Wait until next season when you'll be looking for ways to get back in shape. But if you have cross country skied a few times or have done some downhill skiing, then the early part of your pregnancy is a good time to gear up and go. The "how-to's" of the sport are relatively easy. If you can walk, you can run — if you can run, you can cross country ski! Let's see how.

Equipment

Getting the hang of skiing is easy and enjoyable if you have the proper equipment.

► *Bindings*
There are two basic binding systems: NNN (New Nordic Norm) and SNS (Salomon Nordic System). Ski boots must match the binding type. You may want to look for a "step-in" binding that eliminates the need to bend over to attach.

Older styled three-pin bindings (Nordic Norm), with or without cables, are still used by backcountry and telemarking enthusiasts.

► *Boots*
Select a boot that feels comfortable. You will want a low cut, light boots for classical skiing. Freestyle boots are higher and offer more support for skating. There are combi-boots as well as skis which are designed for both striding and skating.

► Skis

Proper ski length depends on your size, skiing ability, and type of skiing you want to do. As a rule, classical skis should reach your wrist when your arm is raised overhead while freestyle skis will be shorter. For classical skiing you need to decide whether you want waxless or waxable skis. "No-wax" skis are popular with recreational skiers — just step onto the ski and go. The downside is that you lose glide and speed. Waxable skis can be "fine-tuned" to the snow conditions by applying different types of wax. Wax under the boot area of the ski provides the grip on the snow allowing you the traction to "kick" or push off. You apply glide wax to the tips and tails of the skis for striding and to the entire ski for skating. A new generation of waxes has simplified both kick and glide waxing but waxable skis still take much more attention.

► Poles

Base your pole length on your height and on the type of skiing you will be doing. Make sure that your poles are not too short. Most good poles have a "right" and "left." The pole generally comes up to your shoulders for striding and for skating the "mustache rule" applies. (The top of the pole reaches the point between your mouth and nose.) The longer length gives you more power throughout the glide.

Visit a shop that specializes in nordic skiing gear. Take an experienced ski friend with you when you're shopping for equipment and ask questions. Look for "ski package" bargains as well as sales at the start and the end of the season. Consider renting equipment or borrowing a friend's set before buying cross country ski equipment.

Technique

As I noted earlier, if you have not cross country skied before, wait until after your pregnancy to start. Here are some technique tips that you can use then, or before your pregnancy.

► Classic

The classical technique is the heart and soul of cross country skiing. Striding in set tracks is the easiest way to learn the fundamentals. To begin, start walking on your skis and let your arms swing naturally, keeping your poles slanted backward. Get a rhythm going. Once you feel comfortable walking on your skis, try jogging. Push off with one foot and drive the other leg forward. <u>The key is the glide.</u> You want to transfer your weight onto the gliding ski completely and "ride the glide." Keep your knees slightly bent and centered over your ski as you put pressure on your heel and bring your other ski ahead. Keep your strides short at first.

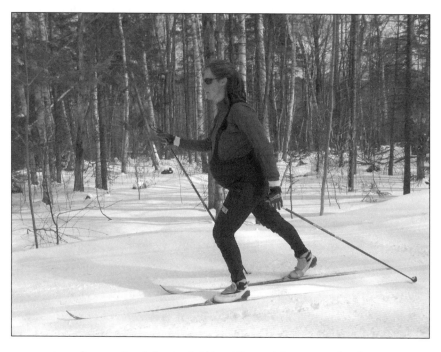

A good example of classical skiing. Her weight is over the ski, the knee is bent, and the ski pole is planted in the snow.

Practice without your poles. This forces you to concentrate on transferring your weight completely and to avoid the common errors of straddling between two skis or using the poles as crutches. Exaggerate your arm swing as you move along. Classical skiing is like running — your right arm comes forward with your left leg. Keep a relaxed grip on your poles and keep the pole tips pointed backward a bit. When your arm comes forward, set the pole tip in the snow and give a little push — this is when you "plant" the pole. Keep your arms slightly bent, plant the pole in the snow and push as you drive past it. One of the best ways to learn, or to improve, is to shadow an experienced skier and mimic his or her movements. Consider taking a few lessons to master the technique. Soon enough, you'll be out on the trail enjoying one of winter's popular pastimes.

► *What About Skating?*

Skating or freestyle skiing is faster than classical skiing and lots of fun. You can skate on open trails, like snowmobile trails, where the packed snow provides a smooth gliding surface. Groomed trails will often have a set of tracks running parallel to a packed trail for skating. Skating on skis requires you to transfer your weight from ski to ski in rhythmic body shifts.

Proper weight transfer and balance are the keys to successful skating. Beginners have trouble "committing" to the gliding ski and instead straddle in between their skis, losing momentum. As you glide, try to align your body (head, hip, and knees) right over the flat ski. A flat ski is a fast ski. Just before starting the next glide, your recovery leg should move in close to your glide leg. At the same time, edge your gliding ski and push off. As the thrusting phase ends, your next gliding phase is beginning on the other leg. Practice by following a good skier, concentrating on shifting weight from ski to ski. Skating without poles can help you master the process.

If you are an experienced skier, there is no reason for you to stop skating while you are pregnant — just watch your intensity level. If you are a novice, better stick with classical technique this season and give freestyle skiing a try next year.

For more information on choosing equipment or for learning technique, there are several excellent books and videos listed in the Resource section.

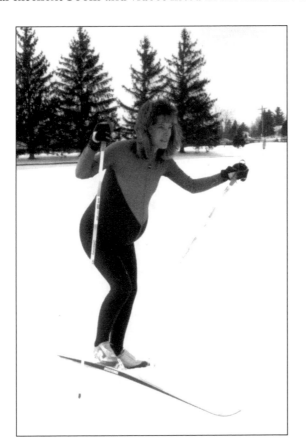

Freestyle is a good option for experienced skiers.

A former Alpine ski racer, Carol, pursued a variety of athletic activities before her three pregnancies. She raced canoes, competed in triathlons (swimming, cycling and running or running, cycling and paddling in a canoe) and cross country skied. She ran and cross country skied throughout all of her pregnancies. For two of her pregnancies, she participated in a study on exercise in pregnancy. "The support system of both the other study participants and the research doctor helped me to better understand my changing body and encouraged me to continue running."

Whitney has been skiing and racing in Vermont since she was 5 years old. She started in her back yard and then joined a Bill Koch league as a youngster. She has been skiing competitively ever since, placing among the top finishers in 25 and 50K races. Whitney has a background in telemark, back country, and cross country skiing, but has focused on the latter. She now coaches high school cross country skiing. Whitney shares her ski routine prior to giving birth to her daughter, a mid-winter baby.

"During pregnancy, I ran until four months, biked until seven months, and dry land trained by hiking and walking. I also continued yoga classes until the end of the 8th month. I wanted to keep up my strength and flexibility. We had a snow drought, so I didn't do a lot of skiing, but everyday I was outdoors for at least an hour exercising.

Initially, skating was more enjoyable than classic skiing because it felt good to go faster than a waddle. I stayed on rolling loops and avoided uphills, though when I did ski uphill, I did so leisurely and relaxed and stopped often to prevent rapid breathing. I was very conscious of my heart rate and I seldom skied more than 5 km. I enjoyed the excursions, but was wary of overdoing it. I fell only twice, in powder, and I wasn't worried at all although the people around me were horrified. My midwife said I was padded and that the baby was well protected. I didn't take chances, but I did love the speed of downhills, especially during pregnancy, because it felt great to go fast. Near the end of pregnancy, I enjoyed classic skiing more, especially since I used no wax skis with automatic bindings to snap into. I felt a lot of pressure in my groin after skiing, so I would immediately go home, put my feet up, and nap.

I was coaching a race the night before I went into labor. It was 10 below in Newport, Vermont. I was warm in a Carhart overall suit and thick boots with toe warmers. The cold and the fun kept me preoccupied and happy. I also think standing on my feet all night may have had something to do with early labor."

Skiing During Pregnancy

► Ski Touring

Touring is basically walking along at a moderate pace on skis. Except for steep hills or deep snow conditions, your rate of perceived exertion will probably stay in the "fairly light" (10 to 12 on RPE scale) zone. Ski with people who match your ability. Nothing is more frustrating than struggling to keep up with an energetic pacesetter — someone who has forgotten that the enjoyment is in the journey, not the miles covered. Set your own pace and take frequent water and rest breaks. Plan a tour that has options if you decide that you want to shorten the outing. A tour in the woods with your partner is a pleasant way to spend an afternoon, get some exercise, and enjoy the outdoors.

► Classical Technique

Classical skiing is safe for both the novice and advanced skier during pregnancy. As you know, your center of gravity and sense of balance has changed. You will need to make some minor adjustments to your technique, like shortening your stride a bit, in the later months. You may find waxless skis a better choice in pregnancy so that you can just put them on and go. Look for step-in bindings to keep it simple to get ready. Obviously your pace will be slower and you will want to avoid steep or rugged terrain. Stay in the 12 to 14 zone on the RPE scale. You may experience mild Braxton Hicks contractions while skiing. Slow down or stop and rest.

> Lisa, a competitive runner, cross country skier, and triathlete found that cross country skiing was a lot easier than running during her pregnancy. Her running pace slowed a bit but not so with skiing. She skied for the first fours months of her second pregnancy before the season ended.

► Skating

As noted earlier, if you are an experienced skier, you will probably enjoy skating on skis during pregnancy. As you might imagine, you will be aware of your added weight as you shift from ski to ski — much more so than in striding. Shortening your glide and skiing on flatter surfaces will help. Skating is a more vigorous workout so avoid long steep uphills. You may need to switch to classical skiing in the last trimester if fatigue or lower abdominal pressure makes skating uncomfortable.

Wendy, an accomplished skier and racer felt like she had "bad wax" while skating at six months pregnant. "It was difficult to move my body into good skating form," she said. "It seemed like an awful lot of work, especially on the uphills."

► *Indoor Skiing*

Indoor ski machines, such as those made by NordicTrack, are another option when skiing conditions are poor or as a year-round workout option. Be sure to exercise in a cool room and drink plenty of water.

► *Ski Racing*

A few cross country ski racers I spoke with raced in the first trimester. However, these women were all well-conditioned athletes, and they avoided overexertion. When I skied (not raced) the tourathon at five months, I kept a steady, relaxed pace. I drank plenty of fluids and snacked along the way. I was prepared to stop at anytime and paid close attention to my body signals. I remember feeling some mild back soreness near the end of the race which went away as soon as I got my skis off.

Snowshoeing

One manufacturer of snowshoes advertises: snowshoes are four-wheel drive for the feet. The new generation of aluminum and neoprene snowshoes is light and easy to use.

Snowshoeing has become more and more popular and can be a good winter activity during pregnancy. You can enjoy the snowy landscape and don't need to have the skills of a skier. The "four-wheel drive" security is perfect when you have a changing center of gravity. Adjustable length poles help your balance and give you a good overall workout.

People often say about snowshoeing, as people did for cross country skiing, "If you can walk, you can snowshoe." It's true: no lessons are required to get out and snowshoe. There are a couple of technique tricks to keep in mind: When climbing a steep hill, push the front of the shoe into the snow first, engage the cleat, and push down. Make it like climbing a ladder. When descending, go heel first, setting the cleat to grip the snow.

Snowshoeing can be strenuous in deep snow and rugged terrain. Stay on easy trails and let your partner and others break trail. Drink plenty of fluids and plan rest stops.

There is no better way to experience the solitude of the winter countryside, and get a nice workout while doing so, than exploring on a modern pair of snowshoes. If you are not an experienced skier or skater, a set of brightly-colored hi-tech snowshoes may be the winter activity that fits you best during your pregnancy.

Pregnancy Tips For Winter Outings

Clear bright skies and sharp temperatures bring joy to the heart of those who like to get some exercise in winter. Don't be tempted to hibernate in the winter and wait for spring just because you are pregnant. Outdoor activity in fresh air is a good antidote for nausea and fatigue in the first trimester of your pregnancy. Even novices will enjoy the safe, low impact workout of cross country skiing or snowshoeing for at least part of pregnancy.

► *Clothing*

If you are a winter exerciser, you already know of the importance of proper dress. Cold temperatures and wind chill can lead to hypothermia (heat loss) and frostbite when you are exercising outdoors. It is even more important during your pregnancy to dress appropriately and think ahead to the conditions you might encounter.

Make sure that you dress in layers (How many times have you heard that?) Layers trap warm air and keep you warmer. For ski touring — which is much like a hike in the woods — and for snowshoeing, three layers works best. The first layer is thermal underwear — the new polypropylenes are great "wickers" of moisture. A comfortable, supportive bra is important. Lycra® tights provide some added support to your lower abdomen, but you may like the feel of a prenatal abdominal support. These are available through mail order, or you can ask your health care provider.

Next, try a turtleneck or light fleece top followed by wind-resistant coat and pants. If you get too warm you can wrap the jacket around your waist. The elastic waist band on the pants should accommodate your abdomen. (You can always borrow a bigger size from your partner or friend.) For more strenuous skiing like striding or skating, you might want to wear tights over thermal underwear. Two pairs of socks, a light poly sock under a wool sock will keep your feet warm and dry. Hats and gloves are crucial — a bare head can throw off 25 per cent of your body heat. You can take gloves off as you heat up and then put them back on as needed. I prefer mittens because of cold hands. Wear sunscreen and sunglasses if it's bright and sunny.

Dress for snowshoeing as you would for nordic skiing — in layers. Wear a comfortable warm pair of boots and bring along a pair of poles. Wear wind pants or a pair of gaiters to keep your legs dry.

► *Hydration*

You may, because of the inconvenience of finding restrooms in the chilly outdoors, be tempted to skip a pre-exercise drink of water. Don't! Even though you may not be perspiring heavily, you still need replacement fluids. Every time you breathe you are losing fluids (respiration). You may notice this in very cold weather when your face mask, scarf, or hat is covered with frost and ice. Carry a fanny pack (or backpack if a fanny pack won't fit around your abdomen) with water and light snacks if you plan to be out for a while. Sip water along the trail. Wear a mini-pad if leaking urine is a problem.

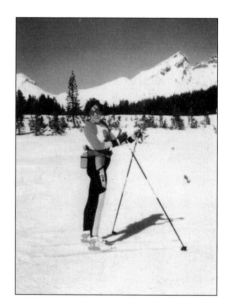

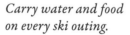
Carry water and food on every ski outing.

► *Where To Ski*

Since we rely on nature and not snowmakers for most nordic skiing, you obviously need to go where there's snow. Ski touring centers offer some advantages. The trails are usually groomed and graded according to difficulty. Restrooms and a place to warm up are usually available, as well as instruction and first aid. Golf courses, local parks, or snowmobile trails are other options. Be familiar with the area, bring along a map if possible, and never ski alone.

► *When To Stop*

You will need to listen to your body to decide when it is time to switch to another activity or to reduce your outdoor winter activities. As one athlete said, "Let your body tell you how much is O.K. but recognize that some pregnancies require restrictions in activity."

Certainly, if you develop any medical complications (see Chapter 3), then you will need to restrict or eliminate skiing and snowshoeing. Keep your health care provider updated on your skiing activities and how you are feeling. If all is going well, you can continue a moderate level of these winter activities, while paying attention to hydration and rest, right up to delivery. Stop if you have pain, bleeding, leaking water, dizziness or other warning signs.

Other winter exercise activities such as downhill skiing, snowboarding, ice skating and sledding are generally too risky during pregnancy due to the possibility of falls. However, if you are suffering from cabin fever and need exercise, a brisk walk is an option in all but the worst weather. So get out there and give that Baby On Board some good fresh winter air.

"At my two-week follow-up visit after my second child, I asked if it was okay to run again. I had stopped running at 3-4 months due to discomfort and had taken up other exercise. I remember that my midwife was surprised that I already felt that I had the time and desire to be out running. But for me, running was freedom – freedom of movement and freedom from mothering, even for a quick 30 minutes." Runner and mother of two

Chapter 13

Delivery and Postpartum

Each woman's pregnancy and delivery will be different. There are many contributing factors, some of which are beyond our ability to influence. So it follows that the delivery experiences of active women are as varied as the women themselves. Being physically active and fit will not guarantee you a fast, painless, and problem-free delivery. The only consistent findings for women who exercised both before and during their pregnancies is that they tend to tolerate labor better. Whitney, skier and mother of Kata Fe, describes her experience:

"My midwives and doctor told me and my husband that some competitive athletes have difficult labors because they compare the labor to a race. They try to stay in control the whole time and this could lead to difficulties. What was so funny was that I was thinking exactly along those lines. I planned to pace myself, keep my body strong and flexible, and in my mind this was going to be the ultimate marathon. Once I spoke with my midwives, I did realize how important it would be to just let go and go with the flow. Although you can prepare for pregnancy, you cannot predict how it is going to happen. Labor and birth was the most intense and incredible experience. The pains were difficult to control or describe. I am very glad that I taught myself to relax and stay happy at all costs. My husband and I stayed together during the whole 21 hours of labor, 3 of those hours were delivery. I only swore once and I did not get angry with my husband. I think that helped. We were a team and it felt so good to be so focused on positive energy."

Woden, runner and mother of three, describes her deliveries:

"Being an athlete influenced my childbirth experience in both positive and negative ways. For me, running has given me an enormous faith in my body. I really looked forward to labor, and I don't remember any fears about birth. I knew my body would do what it was meant to do. Working with a midwife and choosing a homebirth were the normal, obvious choices – and those choices, more than anything else, made my three labors and births the most transcendent experiences in my life.

I do think that first labors can be surprisingly hard for women athletes. First, my frame of reference was all wrong. I was – I admit it – cocky. I imagined labor as being like a marathon or an ultramarathon. I knew it would be hard, but I knew I could handle hard. The reality shocked me. Labor is an experience like no other.

Second, labor requires a different kind of response than the kind of self-discipline I knew as an athlete. From running, I was used to meeting pain head-on: gritting my teeth and pushing through. I tried this in my first labor, and found myself exhausted, frustrated, and totally overwhelmed – at one cm dilation. I knew it was going to get infinitely harder and had no idea how I was going to make it. In the course of that labor, I had to learn how to meet the pain of contractions in an entirely different way: not trying to control them, not focusing on the goal, but instead being present and letting these cosmic forces work through my body. It is an incredible metaphor for motherhood."

Here are the labor experiences (and the baby's weight) of some of the women I interviewed. See how they felt their fitness affected their delivery. (Baby's name and birth weight follows each quote.)

What Others Say

"Exercising regularly kept me focused during labor. I believe being in shape helped with the last stage. I had the energy to continue as labor progressed." (Samuel, eight pounds, three ounces)

"I had good control and strength. I breathed through my labor (6 hours) the same way I did lifting weights." (Taryn, eight pounds, twelve ounces)

"I was induced with Pitocin® because I was overdue. I had hard labor for four hours and then pushed for two hours. I think exercise gave me more endurance but may have made my pelvic muscles tight." (Justin, eight pounds, five ounces)

"My first labor was 19 hours. My second labor was 38 hours total — 12 were hard labor. I had expected an easy labor since I was "fit" but found it wasn't the case." (Daniel, eight pounds, nine ounces)

"Labor with my first was so intense. It began with pains a few minutes apart and continued through the night and morning. I pushed for about 3 hours before receiving a C-section. This takes an enormous amount of strength." (Travis, eight pounds, eight ounces)

"I could concentrate on the rhythm of my body without fear, especially when pushing for all my labors." (Sarah, seven pounds, two ounces; Forrest, seven pounds, two ounces; and Lillian, six pounds, ten ounces)

"I was tired during the labor because I had run that morning and climbed a mountain the day before, but I never had any real difficulty. Perhaps exercise taught me endurance and 'toughness.'" (Stella, eight pounds)

"I was fit so my recovery was very good. My first labor was the same length as one of our longer canoe races." (9 hours) (Vickie, eight pounds, nine ounces)

Now that your nine-month journey has ended with the welcome birth of your baby, you and your partner are beginning a new stage of labor — life with baby. If you kept fit during pregnancy, you are probably eager to "get it back" and resume an exercise program. Fortunately, for most fit women, it won't take another nine months to recover and get back your shape. But, before you get started, take a moment to reflect on the tremendous changes your body has gone through over the past nine months: the rigorous muscle stretching, the ligament and joint laxity, the increased blood volume and hormone surges, to name just a few. Now, your body is beginning the process of returning to its pre-pregnancy state. Let's first take a look at some of these postpartum physical and emotional changes, and then we'll talk about resuming an exercise program.

Physical Changes — Pregnancy In Reverse

Your uterus, that amazing muscular bag, grew from three and a half ounces to nearly 2.2 pounds in weight. It will begin contracting, a process known as "involution," shortly after your baby's birth. These contractions, or "after pains," occur naturally and can be stimulated by breastfeeding. Your uterus returns to its normal size by about six weeks postpartum. Expect bleeding after birth lasting from two to four weeks. However, if your bleeding suddenly gets heavier, this may be a warning sign that you're doing too much and need to slow down.

Your pelvic floor muscles, the muscles that support your uterus, bladder, and rectum, were stretched while you were pregnant and during the delivery of your baby. If you had stitching for a large tear or episiotomy, expect the area to be sore for several days. You can sit in a warm shallow bath to get relief and to promote healing. Keep the area clean and dry. There's also a good chance that the leaking of urine may have been a problem near the end of your pregnancy and may continue now. Kegel exercises, which hopefully you practiced during pregnancy (by contracting the muscles around your vagina), will strengthen these important muscles and speed up the healing process of an episiotomy or repair.

Your abdomen — the focus of so much attention for the last nine months — is again the focus of your attention as you gaze at what probably looks like a loose bulge of flesh. You were hoping, I'm sure, that once the baby was out, you would regain a flat stomach again. It's going to take a little work for that to happen. I'll describe some exercises later in the chapter.

Your abdominal rectus muscles (the two up and down muscles) had the awesome task of stretching around your growing uterus. Diastasis recti, a separation of the muscles, can occur in some women and contributes to lower backache. It's important to begin abdominal exercises soon after delivery.

If you plan to nurse, get your baby on the breast as soon as possible. Your breasts will begin to leak colostrum, the pre-milk liquid that provides nourishment and antibodies. Your milk comes in by the third or fourth day postpartum. Frequent nursing and a good supportive bra will help relieve any engorgement. Wear a tight, supportive bra and apply ice packs if you are not nursing and your breasts become engorged.

Lower back pain is one of the most common complaints in pregnancy and postpartum. It is important that you practice good posture and proper back care from day one.

Posture Tips

- Stand tall — head pulled up, shoulders down. Tighten your buttocks and pull in your abdominal muscles.
- Wear a supportive bra.
- When sitting, press your lower back into the back of the chair. Try not to slouch.
- Place your baby on a pillow and rest your feet on a stool when you nurse. This raises the baby closer to you and prevents stooping over the baby. I set up a "nursing chair" with a pillow and small stool.
- Always think of your back when lifting or carrying your baby.
- Make sure stroller handles are long enough for your height (some models have adjustable handles).
- Front baby carriers should hold the baby snugly to your chest and have adjustable straps.
- Lift with bent knees, pull in your abdominal muscles, and tuck in your buttocks.

Emotional Changes — This Too Shall Pass

Giving birth to your baby requires that you go through your own rebirth in a sense. Once your baby leaves your womb, get ready to share what may be the strongest bond you will ever have with another human. That's not to say that this crossing over into parenthood is a non-traumatic step. Each step of the way will challenge you as you experience one of life's most important events. Prepare for some of these emotions and you may be able to cope more easily.

The first few days, weeks, and even months of your baby's life is a period of tremendous adjustment for the baby and for you. Even though you have been "expecting," suddenly, with no time to warm up, you seem to in a new race. The adjustment to a new baby feels overwhelming to many active couples — especially if you are both used to a life of order and routine.

"It's not what babies do to your body — it's what they do to your life." A swimmer and mother of six

A new baby leaves no part of your life untouched. Your routines will be upset, schedules changed, and adjustments made. You may feel that you have no freedom and the responsibilities of parenting feel overwhelming. It's easy to lose your perspective among sleepless nights, a parade of visitors, and dirty laundry. You may feel blissful one minute and agitated or sad the next. What's happening?

The following table gives you an approximate idea of how long it takes for your physiology to revert back to the non-pregnant state:

The Blues

Like many new moms, you may begin to feel low two to three days after your baby is born. Your hormones (estrogen and progesterone) have suddenly dropped after the birth. Lack of sleep and an abundance of new stressors can lead to feeling down, depressed, or

Approximate Recovery Times
- Cardiovascular system - 2 weeks.
- Abdominal tone - 6 weeks.
- Joints & ligaments - 12 weeks plus.
- Lochia (bleeding) - 3 weeks.
- Urinary tract - 8 weeks.
- Episiotomy - 2 weeks.
  Elaine Cooper from *Running Writing*

irritable. Now is the time to be easy on yourself and "take one day at a time." Look over the following suggestions for coping and give them a try. If you find yourself becoming increasingly depressed, don't hesitate to seek help. Talk to your health care provider and get in touch with " Postpartum Support International," a worldwide support group. (http://www.postpartum.net/)

Coping

► *Rest*

The old saying, "rest when your baby naps" still applies. Accept any and all help from friends and family. I can remember how relaxing it felt to sit nursing my son as my mom buzzed around the house tidying up and doing laundry. From the very beginning, use the teamwork approach with your partner. Avoid the tendency to place "ownership" on the baby — doing everything yourself. Remember, it's a twenty-four hour job. Share the duties and be flexible. If you already have other children, make the most of catnaps or sitting down for a breather.

► *Support*

Somehow six weeks has become the landmark for "getting back to normal." For the past nine months, you have practically lived at your practitioner's office, and now, suddenly, you're on your own. If you are returning to work outside the house, you'll add even more to the stress. Be sure to stay connected to family, friends, or other moms who know what you are feeling. Share your feelings with your partner and try to get some "couple time."

► *Nurturing — Your Baby and Yourself*

Caring for your baby is hard work. You need time out and time alone. Exercise is time well spent. It boosts your physical energy as well as refuels the mothering tank. If you are a list maker, stop now. Reviewing a list of undone things at the end of the day will just make you more frustrated. Instead, set some general goals and take advantage of those 15-minute snatches of time in between diapering, feeding, and bathing. I remember thinking how relaxing and restful my eight week maternity leave would be. I had visions of sitting in the yard, blissfully finishing a baby quilt I had started as my baby lay napping next to me. Guess what? The baby quilt is still not done two years later.

For Dads

You too are going through your own emotional passage. For nine months you watched and waited. Now, with your baby's arrival, you have the opportunity to learn about yourself as a father, partner, caregiver, and child-raiser. Right from the start, a hands-on approach is best. The more you do, the closer you will feel toward your child. Much of the early bonding to a baby comes with simply participating in the care and everyday (and night) routines. These early bonds are strong and provide the foundation for a healthy family.

Appreciate the tremendous physical and emotional changes your partner is going through. Patience is key. Give some leeway for the moodiness. Listen to her concerns and try to offer support. Maybe you need to put some of your needs on temporary hold. Give her the chance to go out for a run, walk, or paddle so she can return refreshed and feeling better about herself. This gives you the opportunity to spend time alone with your baby. The first few weeks are a period of incredible readjustment for both of you.

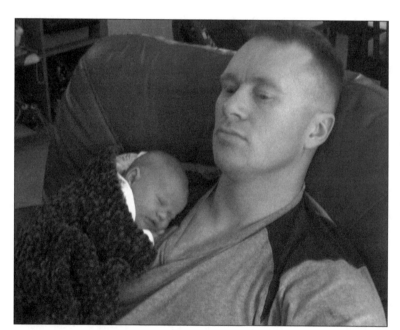

A new baby leaves no part of your life untouched.

Early Exercises

Whether your labor was long or short, vaginal or Cesarean, you can begin some simple exercises in the first few days. You are probably eager to jump back on your bike or go out for a jog. Hold on. Your muscles and connective tissue need time to regain strength and tone. Your joints and ligaments are vulnerable to injury, so you should avoid any jarring activities initially. For now, focus on your abdomen and pelvic floor muscles. Practice proper breathing techniques and stop if you feel any pain. Check with your health care provider before starting.

► *Easy Abdominals*

Lie on your back with knees bent, take a slow deep breath and, as you exhale, tighten your abdominal muscles. Try to hold the contraction for a count to five. Do ten repetitions a day.

Stay lying on your back with knees bent and feet flat. Press your back into the floor and slide your legs away from you while keeping your back pressed downward. Take a breath in, blow out, and slowly slide your feet back. Start slowly and build up to ten repetitions.

► *Kegels*

Your pelvic floor muscles need exercise even if you had a Cesarean. Concentrate on tightening the muscles around your vagina and hold for a count of 8 to 10. You can do this exercise anytime, anywhere. Work up to 25 repetitions during the day.

► *Pelvic Tilt*

This is a great exercise for good posture and relief from backache. Lie on your back with knees bent and exhale as you press your lower back into the floor and hold for a count to ten. Now inhale and relax. You can also do this standing while pressing the small of your back into the wall. Do ten repetitions a day.

Later Exercises — Getting It Back

Very little information currently exists about exercise during the postpartum period and during breastfeeding. One thing is certain, if you were active and fit during your pregnancy, you should be able to resume a gradual program before your six-week checkup. Most physically active women do. But just like during pregnancy, you need to individualize your exercise program and discuss it with your health care provider. Your postpartum fitness goals are to heal, stay healthy, and start back gradually.

If you had an uncomplicated vaginal birth, you can probably start an <u>easy</u> program at about two weeks postpartum. Be aware of joint and ligament laxity which can last several weeks — sometimes up to three months. You'll be more pressed than ever for time but always warm up beforehand, even though it is tempting to skip the warm up and head out the door for your run. Try doing some stretches as you change into your exercise gear or as you are giving last minute instructions to the sitter. Warming up, cooling down, and stretching are integral parts of your workout so allow some time. Drink plenty of liquids, especially if you are nursing. Avoid exercises like cycling or paddling if you had an episiotomy. Wait until you are pain free. Monitor your vaginal bleeding. If it suddenly gets heavier or starts up again, you need to back off and do less. So what <u>can</u> you do?

Whether you had a vaginal or Cesarean birth, give yourself a week or so off and then ease back into exercise with easy strolls. You'll benefit from the rest and get back to your prepregnancy energy levels faster by resting and then gradually building up the intensity and duration. Enjoy the pleasure of walking with your baby and the opportunity to spend some time with your partner without distractions. At about two to six weeks, if all is going well, you might want to begin low impact aerobics or a special postpartum exercise class. If you had a Cesarean birth, then you need to avoid strenuous abdominal exercises until the inner layer of the incision has healed, usually in 4 to 6 weeks. Following surgery, it's not uncommon to feel some twinges and pulling sensations while exercising. Stop if you feel sharp pain. Wear a pad if leaking urine is a problem and remember: Kegels — Kegels — Kegels!

Here's the candid observation of one mother on her recovery from childbirth:

"I started exercising way too soon after the birth of my first child. I recovered really well and I wanted to be up and doing. I also missed that feeling of freedom running through the woods. So I went out for a short run at the end of the first week postpartum, and kept trying to do more. My body was fine except for my pelvic muscles, which were very weak, so continence was a problem. I was shocked. It was hardly the vision I'd had of myself, loping along like in my old athletic days; instead I was hobbling, breasts enormous with milk, belly jiggling, dribbling all the way. No fun. I'm pretty sure the pounding weakened my pelvic muscles: not only did it take a while to recover, but I had a prolapse after my second baby."

Low intensity stair climbing is another option as well as riding a stationary bike, treadmill walking, cross country skiing, paddling or rowing. All of these activities are low impact and you can easily modify them to suit your mood or energy level. Again, be very cautious of your vulnerable joints and ligaments and keep it light to moderate.

What about swimming? Although swimming is non-impact you should wait to get in the pool until your bleeding has stopped since you will be wearing pads and not tampons. Your Cesarean incision should be entirely healed before resuming swimming so consult your medical provider.

Later, you can gradually integrate more jarring activities like high impact aerobics and running into your program. You can start walking and doing toning exercises with light weights and then work up to jogging or aerobics. Delay serious weight training until about six weeks after the baby. Elite and competitive runners I spoke with gradually started back with light jogging after vaginal deliveries in one to 4 weeks. Many breastfeeding runners commented on the challenge of running with larger or tender breasts.

> Samantha, a yoga instructor and new mom, believes that introducing your children to yoga at a young age gives them a foundation for body awareness and positive self-image as they grow older. Yoga has been known to promote better sleeping, stimulate neuromuscular development, improve colic or gas pains, and build a healthy bond between parent and child, says Samantha. Look for mommy and me yoga classes that are available at certain yoga studios.

Breastfeeding and exercise are very compatible. There is no evidence that exercise will diminish the quality of your milk, and nursing is a real time saver — no bottles or formula to worry about. Plan to nurse your baby right before you exercise, or if it's not time for a feeding, pump your breasts. Get a "megasupport" bra or try wearing two bras. "I went from an A/B cup to an E cup," reported one Olympic runner. Another elite runner would stop to nurse her daughter in the baby jogger while out for longer runs. Use nursing pads if leaking breasts are a problem. I cut up panty liners and stuck them on the inside of my bras. Some nursing moms told me that they felt more tired during the time they were breastfeeding.

Remember the importance of a balanced diet. Depending on your activity level, you need an additional 400 to 500 calories a day and lots of fluids, 10 to 12 glasses. You may hear that exercise will cause your milk to sour due to lactic acid buildup. I wouldn't worry — if you exercise at a moderate level it is unlikely that this will happen. Besides, if you nurse before exercise you will avoid any such possibility.

Fit women like yourself are anxious to "get it back" — the fitness — but are just as anxious to "get it off" — the weight. After delivery, you will lose the weight of the baby, the placenta, and fluids, but you still will be heavier than you were before you became pregnant. But, since you are coping with so many things already, don't be concerned about weight loss for now. If you are not nursing, you can begin a sensible weight loss program. However, skimping calories is not wise, especially during the first six weeks when you need energy and stamina. A program of exercise and breastfeeding is no guarantee for weight loss in itself. Most active nursing mothers gradually lose the weight without really trying. But, it's not uncommon to carry a few extra pounds until you wean the baby. Follow a well-balanced diet (See Chapter 4) and be sure to get enough calcium, about 1200 mg. a day, according to RDA guidelines.

Whether you breast feed or not, take your time and be sensible as you move toward your prepregnancy weight. If you are not nursing, you may have started birth control pills for contraception. Some women claim that it is harder to lose weight while taking birth control pills. This has not been scientifically proven, especially with the newer low dose pills. Regardless of whether you nurse or bottle feed, or take hormonal methods of contraception or not, try to create a healthy balance of diet, exercise, and rest.

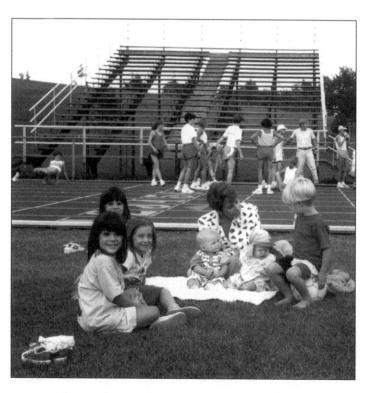

Babies and kids relax while moms get ready to run.

Competition ... When To Start

I read an article in a running magazine which suggested wearing a weighted vest during training. The theory was that the added weight would increase leg-muscle power and speed without doing any special workouts. I couldn't help but think of pregnancy as a built-in "training vest." Does pregnancy make you a better athlete?

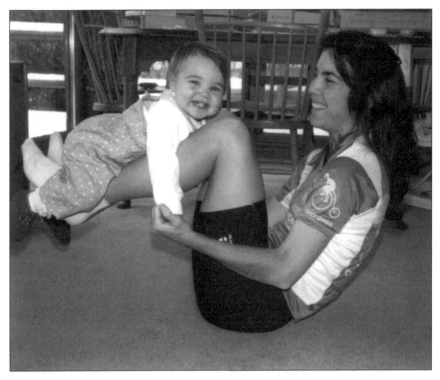

Getting back to your pre-pregnancy shape and stamina is important but also very individual.

There are no studies to confirm if the physiological changes in pregnancy enhance athletic performance. Psychologically, there may be a positive effect. Track stars like Ingrid Kristiansen, Valerie Brisco, and Tatyana Kazankina all took their performance to new levels following their pregnancies. Ireland's Sonia O`Sullivan ran during both of her pregnancies. She was third in the 2002 World Cross Country 4k Championships only three months after the birth of her second child. Valerie Brisco won two gold medals in the 1984 Olympics two years after having her son. Two years after her daughter's birth, Susan Notorangelo won the women's RAAM (Race Across AMerica) race.

Many competitive athletes have said that pregnancy, particularly labor, enhanced their mental and emotional stamina. For example, five months after delivery, Ingrid

Kristiansen ran her fastest marathon — which she then improved upon the next year. She credits her family interests with helping her become a better runner. Other athletes agree. When you're a mother, you tend to use your training time more efficiently. You become more focused.

If you are an elite or professional athlete, you likely had special supervision of your pregnancy by your health provider. You probably, with luck, were able to plan your pregnancy during an off-season. Most of the elite athletes I spoke with had just finished a vigorous racing season and were planning to get pregnant. One professional runner decided to get pregnant due to a broken foot. A competitive canoe racer went all out in the season previous to trying to get pregnant and placed second in the National Championships. "I wanted to do well because I didn't know when my next chance to race would be." Another marathon canoe racer conveniently had both her babies in December. She nursed and recovered during January through April and then started racing again in May. If you're like most active women I spoke with, you fit your athletic pursuits in around your pregnancy and the birth of your child — not the other way around.

Your return to competition is individual and dependent on your delivery experience and recovery. Regaining your prepregnancy fitness level takes time, and for some women, may never happen. Some competitive runners took one to two years to get it back. One 35-year-old Olympic runner began racing after seven months but was plagued by fatigue and frequent viral infections. She realized that she was doing too much, too soon. She backed off and waited several months before racing again. After 21 months she clocked a 20:40 for a 4 mile race and later a 33:06 in a competitive 10K race. A former Olympic rower and mother of three returned to competition at three months and set a personal indoor record ten months later. She felt that her pregnancies did not provide a training effect, but being a mother brought a "focus effect" to her training. The time she does have to train is more intense and higher quality.

Whether you are a national-class athlete or an "around-the-block" jogger, you'll find that getting back to your pre-pregnancy shape and stamina is important but also very individual. Don't compare yourself to others or expect a miraculous comeback. The key to successful recovery is moderation, going slowly, and listening to your body. Remember, your body signals guided you through your pregnancy, and they will help you safely recover and get fit.

"The big thing is putting off the dishes and laundry and all that other stuff and fitting exercise in when I can, and making it a top priority. I'm lucky to live in a town where I can walk so much and to have a supportive husband who believes my fitness and well being are as important to the family as they are to me." Mother of two

Chapter 14

Life After Baby - The Fit Family

Parenthood, as you are learning, is an on-going, ever-changing enterprise. Each day has new surprises, joys, obstacles, and challenges. You and your partner are discovering the realities of family life. No book or class can prepare you for life with your baby. In no time at all, you won't remember what life was like without your baby.

For many of you, returning to work is the next phase of adjustment. Safe, reliable childcare is the cornerstone to the functioning of working families. Whether in your home, private home, or day care center, the best childcare is what suits your family's needs. If your child is in a safe and happy care setting, you and your partner can begin to develop some strategies for fitting in exercise. But how?

Parenting is an elemental lesson in time management. You feel as if you have more and more to do and less and less time to do it. The key to survival is setting priorities and keeping your expectations in line. (Aim for the gold but settle for silver.) Now is the time for you and your partner to honestly discuss your fitness goals. Do you want to exercise for general fitness, weight loss, or competition? How many hours (or minutes) per day are "yours?" What options do you have to fit in 30 minutes — an hour a day? Do you prefer to exercise alone, with a buddy or in a class? If your partner is also active, how do your goals mesh?

Woden, mother of three, changed her sports.

"The thing I miss most in my life as a mother is my daily run. If I could add one thing, that would be it. I long for that sense of freedom and the meditative time. Many women find time for this, but our family circumstances are such that it doesn't work for me. I tried running with a baby jogger and found it totally unsatisfying: heavy and confining, far too much of a workout and far too little of the freedom I want from my runs. I've struggled with not running, but have realized that this is such a brief moment in my life – my kids are 3, 2 and 1 – and those trails will be there when I am ready to go back to them.

What I do instead is league sports: soccer and broomball. The games are 1-2 times a week, and they're at night so Mark is home. Because my teammates need me, I have to go, even when I really just want to fall into bed. It's great. I show up, run like crazy for an hour, and get that sense of exhilaration. Plus I love the sense of toughness that comes from playing broomball – with all its pushing and penalties -- over and against the fragility I often feel as a mother."

Fitting It All In

Whether you are at home with your child (children) or working outside, finding time to exercise is a challenge. Perhaps you are home with two or three young children or your job requires travel or long hours, or both you and your partner are competitive athletes. Finding time to exercise while balancing family and work is not easy, but many active families are doing it. Here are some comments from a few:

What Others Say

"I am able to maintain a fairly good balance between family, work, exercise because I am not driven to be the best at everything. I'm willing to sacrifice some things, like a perfectly clean house, for a chance to take Rebecca for a walk or go for a bike ride." (A cyclist.)

"Having kids has greatly reduced my opportunities for consistent exercise. Now that I am out of the habit of regular exercise, it is hard to get as motivated as I once was. My priorities are my family and home. Work is necessary, and exercise, while important, is difficult to fit in." (A marathon canoe racer.)

"With age and family I've gotten wiser about my training. I made a choice to stay home with my two children because I want to spend time with my family. A stationary bike, rowing machine, baby jogger, and pulk for skiing, as well as a cooperative husband all help me stay fit." (A cross country skier, triathlete.)

"Competition no longer seems like a priority as it once was. However, overall fitness is. I look at exercise as general body maintenance, like daily personal hygiene. (A runner, triathlete, marathon canoe racer.)

"My priorities are very clear in my mind. My career has always been very important but I don't believe it requires 60-80 hours a week, and it doesn't make me as happy as my son does. Also, I manage stress at work much better when I'm exercising regularly." (A swimmer.)

(From a dad) "I continued to train and race throughout my wife's pregnancy; however, I think the intensity of my training decreased because I lacked her as a training partner. The racing and training became lower in significance. After our daughter was born, we were fortunate to have good friends who would baby-sit during periods that we wanted to train. When my wife got back into competition, my motivation and training improved." (A marathon canoe racer and cross country skier.)

Goals

What are your fitness goals now that the baby is here? Many women I spoke with found that their competitive drive was diminished after having children. Training for competition requires a substantial time and mental commitment. It's natural that your priorities will change. Being fit and feeling good about yourself are important but may pale in comparison to the importance of your role as a parent. Parenthood may be an opportunity to move out of competition and continue your sport for fun — or to take up a new sport(s).

On the other hand, some women are fired up to get back into competition following their pregnancies. Returning to competition gives you goals to strive for in your training program.

> An Olympic runner noted, "I have a supportive husband, a wonderful baby sitter, and a strong desire to race again at the same or higher level!"

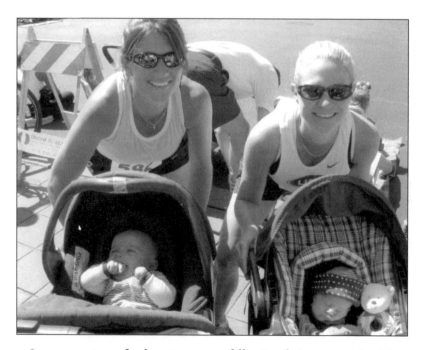

Some women are fired up to compete following their pregnancies. The mom on the left won the 5K race when her son was three months old.

Most of us will have a new perspective on exercise after having a child. Here, a former downhill ski racer and triathlete explains how her exercise goals changed with parenthood.

"My three-year-old points to the front of my T-shirt and asks", 'What's that, Mommy?'

'That's a narwhal. This shirt was for Mom's swim team in Alaska, back when I used to get exercise.'

"I catch myself. Here I am walking down a trail in the woods, with the legs of my thirty-plus-pound son wrapped around my waist and my hands around his back, holding him in this conversational position. In my backpack, my twenty-pound one-year-old is jumping and leaning, trying to reach her brother's face and using my hair for extra balance. We've been walking this way for ten minutes and have at least five more to go. And I feel like I don't get any exercise?

It's funny, I reflect, how we reach our definition of exercise. My "formal training" started when I was eleven when I mowed a one-eighth-mile somewhat oval track in the field in front of our house. Every morning before school I would pop out of bed, don my "run-faster" Keds sneakers and head for the track. The routine set the approach I was to use for the next twenty-five years.

From age ten through college I was a competitive downhill skier. Cross training was part of my personality so I varied my training daily and seasonally. I played field hockey and soccer, ran, lifted weights, went backpacking and biking, and engaged in many other sports. Nearly all my choices involved movement of my entire body and at least twenty minutes of sweat-producing, heavy-breathing exertion — that's what I call exercise.

After a setback from knee surgery, I became involved in competitive triathlons at age thirty. By this time, cross country skiing had become a passion, and I spent the long Alaskan winters with about two hours each weekday on the tracks and weekends telemarking in the backcountry. I balanced that out with long pool workouts, speed hikes of one to two hours with big elevation gains, ocean kayaking, biking, and a non-stop lifestyle.

By age thirty-six, I was back in rural New York, married, and still exercising formally and informally every day. My son was born in September after an active pregnancy of thirty-mile bike rides, firewood cutting and splitting, one-hour lap swims, and a long summer of active farming.

Then the priorities changed. There were still cross country ski outings that winter, but they were slower and shorter with the baby along. Summer bike rides now included scenic stops along the way and a mid-point picnic or exploration. Exercise for its own sake was replaced by easy-going outings with the baby. Quick naps, catching up on the bills, or making those necessary phone calls where I did not want to be distracted by kid noise or tugging, robbed me of those moments where it seemed I would be able to workout on my own.

My lifetime of being in shape carried me along. My upper body and back stayed strong from kid hauling. Our outings were frequent enough to keep my aerobic capacity up. In my few kid-free jaunts with non-parent friends, I was still able to keep up or even surprise them with my physical condition.

Now, with two children, the slow shift from what I still call "exercise" continued. Yet I felt going slower and answering the hundreds of three-year-old questions was more important. At home, I continuously scrambled to stay on top of the basic life maintenance activities like food, dishes, bills, and laundry. My bike wind trainer and yes, even my skis gathered dust.

This bothered me — a lot. But it was my choice. With parenthood, priorities have to be made and I did it this way. In my calmer moments, I consider those years just a different form of training. I kept, and even developed some strong muscles masses. Sleep deprivation and midnight wakings developed discipline to do things I really didn't want to do, and the ability to perform even when dead tired. My endurance was probably better than in my triathlon days, because my kid triathlons were often twelve hours long.

Probably the most important learning of parenting is that whatever you do, if you do it with some thought and conviction, then it is the right thing to do. Someday, I'm sure, I will be able to bike, hike, run, and swim hard again — maybe even competitively. Aerobic exercise will again be my norm. Or will it? I guess I don't dare predict. Whatever happens, it will be right.

Take some time to settle in on your fitness goals as you deal with the new demands on your time. Whether you choose competition or fitness, set some goals that will help you stay challenged and motivated while having fun. A combination of involving your child in sports and still getting some time for independent exercise seems to be the success behind fit families."

Finding The Time

Whitney, cross country skier and mother of one daughter, discusses solo fitness time.

"Fitness to me has changed in its definition. I know my role as a mom comes first. I still do 10 minutes of yoga each morning or night if I can just to stretch out my back and my sore muscles from carrying Kata Fe. I think stretching is more difficult and more important than it has ever been. I definitely make use of my free time between work and getting to daycare. I run, ski or workout with a commitment that I lacked in the past few years because alone time is precious and necessary for my sanity. I am still a happy mom even a year later and our daughter is a healthy outdoors kind of baby."

Whitney also reflects on family ski time with her daughter and husband, former Olympic cross country skier Marc.

"We began hiking with our daughter Kata Fe at about 6 months with a backpack because she'd outgrown the Baby Bjorn. We have skied with her using both a backpack and a ski pulk. She loves the pulk. We are able to ski 15 km without her getting tired. My husband pulls and I am able to keep up at his pace because I am still not in the shape I used to be. We skate because it is a smoother rhythm. I pull her myself when I'm all alone, and I backpack with her often. It is nice to give my husband the extra weight, to slow him down, and try and be equals as I slowly continue to get back in shape."

Suzanne, active runner and mother of three says:

"I have had to go on 10 mile runs pushing two kids in a baby jogger but normally, I get up very early in the morning to get my runs in. But it's not that hard to make it work if you are motivated. The hardest part is finding other people that want to join you that early in the morning!"

Cindy, a mother of three, noted that she's more relaxed about exercise:

"I was pretty burned out on competitive running by the end of college, and as I transitioned to more of a recreational runner I still had feelings that I should be doing more. Now, I make a point of exercising outdoors each day, and although my preference is to run, I often do something else instead. Running seems to be the simplest with kids (it takes the least time and I can just go from home and can bring a kid in the jogger), but I do other things too. In the winter, I tend to drop my mileage (~10-15 miles per week), but then supplement with xc skiing, snow shoeing and ice skating. My running mileage fluctuates quite a bit depending on the season, the stages my kids are at, how chaotic things feel at home, and how much time I can get away, but as long as I can do something outside most every day I am happy. We also try to plan family activities around seasonal outdoor activities... hiking, swimming, skating, xc skiing, and kayaking. We also make a point of walking or biking places (can be tough in a rural area) instead of using the car when feasible. For example, my boys walk about a mile each way to and from school each day."

Change Your Routine
A mother of two says:
"I miss running with my husband. Now, we each take turns and occasionally run together if we arrange child care."

Teamwork

Maintaining fitness in an active family requires a substantial amount of teamwork. There will be days when you will feel as though anarchy has set in and defeat is just around the corner. Keep your perspective, for as they say, there is always tomorrow. You and your partner need to design your own strategies for meeting your baby's needs, doing household chores, and attending to the myriad of details that penetrate your daily lives. Mornings can feel like a strategic planning session as you discuss the day's plans and activities. Hopefully, part of that discussion is when, where, and for how long you will exercise.

A big change for some couples is spending less time training together. The teamwork concept will work if you are both able to share your expectations, and you are able to talk about those expectations. Think ahead, plan ahead and talk about it.

Jan, cyclist and mother of three, explains how it works in her family:

> *"Doug and I try to have our personal time to go on rides, independently or together. The kids love riding so we spend time riding around the yard or going to the bike paths to be able to get out. We recently got a Cannondale tandem and have installed a child's stroller kit so one of the kids can ride in the back. We have gone through the child seats, trailers, helmets, and the all of the sudden the "I am tired" rides with the kids. We are looking forward to many days of riding together and hopefully some touring with the kids."*

Flexibility

Flexibility — parenting gives new meaning to the word. It seems as if plans are always being changed by things like a sick child or a canceled sitter. Try to stay flexible. Look at these "crises" as an adventure in creativity.

Let's look at an example. You planned to run with the running stroller when your baby awakens from her nap. Now it's pouring rain. What are some alternatives? Why not hop on the wind trainer, start up an exercise video, or crank up the cross country ski machine? Use your athletic traits, determination, and fortitude to adapt to the new situations that are constantly arising. As one mother said, "Parenting is a form of cross training."

Sue, a runner and mother of two girls outlines what works for her:

"I have been very fortunate to have a supportive husband and two children that are excited to go to races and watch. I usually run right after work before I pick the kids up from day care. On weekends Joe and I take turns going for our long runs. We used to do these together, but now we have to split it up. Our daughter, Caroline has been running in races sponsored by the Many Miler program and I am sure that in a couple years, her sister Mary will be chasing her around the roads and trails."

How flexible are you — not your joints, but your attitude? An area of debate is whether exercise is a positive or negative addiction. For some of us, the compulsion to exercise can become a negative aspect of staying fit. Missing a workout or having to change plans can bring feelings of guilt or disappointment. Obsessive feelings about exercise can erode the positive benefits such as stress reduction and a sense of well-being. Some of the signs of addiction to exercise are: recurrent overuse injuries, weight loss, resistance to "cutting back," exercising through pain, and neglecting the other areas of your life. Only you know if you are losing the benefits by being too inflexible — by letting exercise assume too much priority and adding more stress to your life and your family.

Patty, a teacher and mother of two, managed to squeeze exercise into her busy schedule:

"Luckily I was able to take time off my teaching job after I had each of my children, so during their infancies I would organize the mornings so that I could run before my husband left for work. When I look back on those days, I remember firmly believing that mornings were the only time I could exercise, but as soon as I returned to teaching I realized I could not be rigid about exercising. I had to be at school by 7:30 A.M. and it is too dark and hazardous to run in the early morning hours, so I learned to become an afternoon runner. Before my children were in elementary school, I would delay picking them up at day care so I could run or I would run just before dinner within the confines of our village. During their pre-teenage years, they participated in various sports and activities so my schedule - and theirs - was even more demanding. I used my "flexible maxim" to find time to exercise. For instance, when I took my daughter to flute lessons I always wore my running clothes and shoes. As soon as she entered her teacher's house, I took off and managed to run for thirty to forty minutes. I followed this same procedure when I took my son to tennis and lacrosse practice. Exercise after children is possible, but it can only be accomplished by being flexible and creative."

Equipment For The Fit Family

Many active families, using teamwork and flexibility, are able to pursue their fitness and even their competitive goals. Fortunately, there is equipment available that will help you take your baby along while exercising. If you're thinking of buying any of these items, talk to someone who owns one and get their feedback. Also, whether it's hiking, cycling, running or skiing, you'll need to do some extra planning for an outing with your baby. Remember the Scout motto, "Be prepared". Anticipate the need to nurse or offer a bottle, and carry spare diapers. Dress your baby warmer than yourself — you're moving and generating heat while your baby is still. Check the weather forecast. Use sun block and hats with a visor for sunny weather. Grab a few toys for entertainment.

Following are descriptions for using a wide range of exercise equipment. See the Resource Section for a sampling of manufacturer's websites.

► *Running Strollers*

There are different styles and models to choose from, and most models fold up for transport. Make sure yours has a braking system (handy when loading and unloading your baby), sturdy tires, and a safety leash in case your baby starts to get away from you. Canopies are handy, and you can also fasten a light towel with clothespins over the front to block sun or wind. It takes some practice running with a stroller. Your stride will shorten and hills can be a real chore. Try to keep a light touch and push with one hand so your other hand can still pump. There are double joggers for twins or your second child. One elite runner told me that she did hill repeats with her two year old and infant in a running stroller. Now that's a workout!

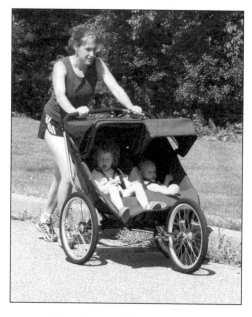

Running strollers are great aids for walking or running.

► *Carriers*

Front carriers are for infants, but once your baby can hold his/her head up, usually at three to four months, you're ready for a back carrier. Try one on with your baby before you buy. Make sure that both the shoulder and waist straps are comfortable. Carriers are great for walking, hiking, a stationary indoor bike, indoor rowing machine, and cross country skiing. We used our backpack for skiing with our son in good weather up until the age of two. Snuggled in the pack, he would usually fall asleep for a nap within the first twenty minutes of the ski. Having this kind of weight on your back requires strength and coordination and should be reserved for shorter outings on relatively flat terrain.

► *Bike Trailers and Child Seats*

Whether riding in a trailer or a child seat, your infant or child must wear a helmet. In some states it's the law — in all states it's common sense. You can put an infant care seat inside the trailer for added neck support. Some trailers also convert to strollers, though a little awkward, and can seat two children (maximum weight 80 to 85 pounds). They come in bright colors and you can place a safety flag on a long pole on the back. You'll find that you can pull bike trailers more easily with a mountain bike. Because a trailer is wider than your bike, avoid congested streets. There are retractable canopies and room in the trailer for snacks and toys.

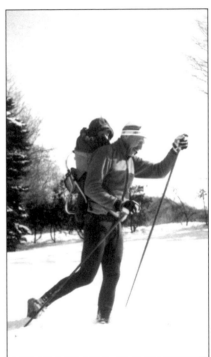

Back carriers work well for cross country skiing.

Child seats are for one year-olds and up. A rear-mounted seat is safer than a front-mount and should have a seat back that isn't so high that it forces your child's head forward. Foot buckets keep toes away from spokes. When mounted, the seat should carry the child's center of gravity ahead of your rear axle. Go to a bike shop if you're not sure about proper mounting. A touring or mountain bike is more stable for carrying a child's seat. Before you launch with your precious cargo, try pulling an empty trailer or riding with a bag of potatoes in the seat. Get used to the added weight and negotiating turns and stopping.

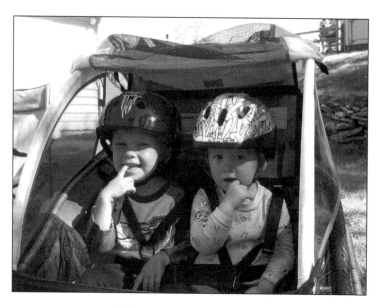

Buckled up and ready to go.

► *Pulk*

A pulk is a ski sled that you can pull while cross country skiing. The sled has runners which glide on groomed ski tracks and is usually pulled by a harness with a waist belt. Some have a shield which protects your child from flying snow and wind. There's plenty of room to pack snacks and extra clothing in the pulk. Remember to bundle up your child and plan outings with "bail out" options if there is a change in weather or mood.

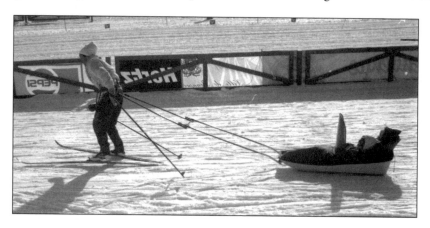

Pulks are popular options at cross country ski sites.

► *Sports Racks*

Car racks come in many designs with added features for lugging bikes, canoes, skis, strollers — you name it. They are a must for family sports outings. Check out the different models and pick one that is compatible with your vehicle and interests.

► Home Fitness Equipment

A home fitness "center" can be as simple as an aerobics tape and hand and ankle weights or as sophisticated as a complete workout room with various workout stations and equipment. It depends on your budget and space limitations. Exercising in your home is backup for inclement weather or for a parent at home without child care arrangements. Getting some exercise in your home is a time saver, and as one mother said, "Something is better than nothing."

► Videotapes/DVD's

There is no lack of variety here — everything from stretching and toning to high intensity aerobics is available. You can simulate a cross country ski, bike ride, or jog as you work out on your machine and visually escape to scenic areas like Switzerland or Hawaii. See the resource section for more information.

► Machines and Workout Equipment

Weight stations, treadmills, steppers, cross country ski machines, rowing machines, stationary bikes, and climbers are all fitness options. Before you buy any piece of equipment, definitely try it out. Get a temporary health club pass and try their equipment to help you decide what you will enjoy and consistently use at home. Look for bargains in the want ads — there is a lot of "slightly used" exercise equipment gathering dust in people's basements. Once you get started, get an iPod® or a flexible belt so that you can wear a CD player. Music will jazz up your workouts on any machine.

Liz is a single parent and works full time. During the first few months after her son was born, she used a NordicTrack® to get back in shape before returning to masters swim workouts. She hires a teen to watch her son during her twice weekly evening swims. She struggles with the emotional conflict of tagging on another sitting arrangement for her son but realizes the benefits she gains from swimming. For Liz, swimming provides her with a period of relaxed concentration. She feels revitalized and ready to engage in the demands of single parenting.

► *Fitness Centers*

The growth of fitness centers is a reflection of the need for time-efficient and versatile exercise options for busy people. Most centers provide one stop shopping for instruction, exercise classes, state of the art equipment, and often, child care. Do your homework before becoming a member. Talk with current members, get a trial pass, and stop by at the time you will most likely use the facility. Are instructors certified? What is the child care like? Talk with other moms. How often will you go? Is it worth the investment? YMCA's or community centers are other options for exercise.

► *Finding Time For Fitness*

One of the biggest impediments to pursuing physical activity is time. When you, or both of you, have been used to freely exercising when you wanted and as long as you wanted, parenting can be a challenging adjustment. If you have two exercise schedules to juggle, it's even more challenging — but not impossible. Communicate, coordinate, and compromise.

For working parents this means examining the demands on your time and coming up with time slots where you can fit in exercise. Before work, during lunch or after work are possibilities. A run or bike ride before breakfast can easily be accomplished while the other person begins the morning routine. Shower facilities at your work place provide the option of cycling or running to work or on your lunch hour. Lunch hour workouts have the advantage of not cutting into time with your family. Fitness centers are another way to squeeze a workout into any of these time slots. Alternate times with your partner for variety. If your family is driving to a nearby destination, throw in a change of clothes in the car, strap on your running shoes and meet them there. Hire a sitter to come along if

> Shelly, a single mother of two small children, tries to balance working full time, the demands of parenting and her desire to maintain her physical fitness. "I'm really forced to be clear about my priorities. I want to spend as much time as possible with my children and at the same time carve out time for some exercise. I think I am able to do this at the expense of social activities." Shelly tries to run during her lunch hour and uses a bike trailer for after work rides in good weather. A vigorous exercise video is an option after her children are settled for sleep. She emphasizes the need to balance exercise with a healthy diet and adequate rest.

you are both competing in an event or take turns competing in different events. Look for races where you have friends or relatives nearby to watch your children. Early on, establish a reliable list of sitters for scheduled exercise plans on weekends.

It requires a bit more creativity if you're home with your child (or children). One mother of two pointed out that "not working outside the home allows more time flexibility but fewer child care options." Take turns with a relative, friend or neighbor watching each other's children. Consider starting a baby-sitting co-op or play group. A health club with child care facilities is a popular alternative. Seize the moments — no matter how brief! Work in a few abdominals, light weights, stretches or jumping rope while your children are involved with an activity. Kids love to join in and copy Mom. Running strollers, bike seats, trailers, and carriers allow you to exercise with your child. The moving motions of any of these pieces of equipment will soothe a cranky baby while you're enjoying the outdoors. Indoor exercise equipment allows you to get a workout during nap times or with your little one in a toy-filled playpen nearby.

Ann, mother of two, tells how she incorporates fitness into her life these days:

"Around the edges! I try to do something, yoga or run or less often, dance, I don't know, 4/5 days out of 7 (whereas before having children I would probably do something every day), but often I'm tired so it isn't necessarily the most inspired workout. But I also go on lots of walks with my now 2 year old, and I do a lot of walking in general because we live in walking distance of most things and, since we live at the top of a very steep hill, so I trust that just walking up that a few times a day is keeping me in good enough shape until I have more time again. Getting exercise is important to me, but so is spending time with my children and getting some work done and so while I do exercise, I'm much more relaxed about it and figure that in a few years it will feel easier and less disruptive to again go for 1 1/2 hour runs, or do long, deep, solitary yoga practices. One interesting shift is that I've started doing authentic movement, a much quieter, more internal and less rigorous form of movement. I think in part because of changes from childbirth and from the experience of having children who have helped me slow down and open to the sweetness of each moment, rather than being so focused on the goal (i.e. how long I am running, etc.)."

Fit Families

Many children today are in trouble due to lack of exercise and poor diet. Many youth watch TV, play video games, and instant message/email several hours a day. Some studies show that fifty per cent exhibit risk factors for heart disease such as high cholesterol and obesity. According to the Centers for Disease Control and Prevention, the percentage of U.S. children and teens (6-19) who are overweight tripled to 16% in the period between 1980 and 2002. There is strong evidence that risks such as obesity in childhood are carried into adulthood.

What's the solution? Encourage physical activity in your children — the sooner, the better. Children who take up physical activities that are fun are healthier, have more self-confidence and self-esteem, a better body image, and a sense of how good it feels to be fit. It's these good feelings that will hopefully carry over into their adult lives as they maintain fitness through a healthy lifestyle.

The best way to get kids motivated and interested in exercise is to set a good example. You may be thinking that you are already being a good role model by running every day and training for your next marathon. Well, that's not enough. We need to participate in activities <u>with</u> our kids that are fun, like swimming, hiking, camping, and sledding, to name a few. Create opportunities for your child to get involved with community recreation programs, sports lessons, and summer camps. Provide the options but let your child choose what he or she <u>wants</u> to participate in. Support their efforts and offer praise along the way.

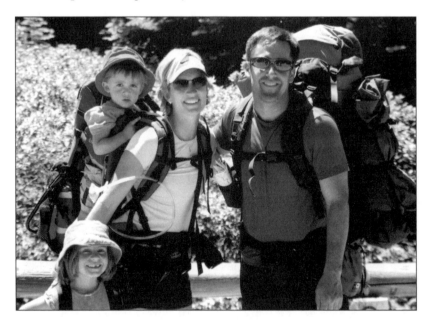

Fun activities like backpacking and camping can teach kids to love outdoor exercise.

If you are a competitive athlete, it's important to emphasize your child's enjoyment and focus less on the "win" mentality. Kids will discover their own competitive drives in due time. What they need most is encouragement and praise for teamwork. They need to be supported as they handle their losses and failures. These are the skills that they will carry over into other areas of their adult lives, in relationships, jobs, and families. Provide children the opportunity to pursue activities they will enjoy when scholastic or collegiate sports are over, activities like hiking, skiing, cycling, or jogging. These and other sports help us return to the basic motivation for all exercise — the sheer pleasure of using our bodies.

A Father's Perspective

I watched my 15-year-old son wrestle in a high school tournament. He came to the match well prepared; he was conditioned, strong and determined — attributes essential to the sport. His participation in athletics goes back to his days as a toddler, when he began skiing, hiking, and canoeing with his parents. He sometimes rode along on his BMX bike while I ran or accompanied me to the weight room while I worked out. Later, when he joined youth soccer, I was the team's coach. He saw me compete in triathlons and cycle and foot races. Today our athletic interests, except for hiking, have diverged: his are scholastic team sports, mine are often solitary conditioning excursions. But we do share a mutual dedication to fitness. It's clear to me that his awareness, his commitment, and his self-motivation were, to a large extent, generated through parental example and shared experiences.

Parent's Perspective

Before we had our children we both enjoyed a very active lifestyle: cross country skiing, hiking and backpacking, running, cycling, paddling canoes, and competing in road races. By doing these physical activities together — in fact, our first "date" was a bike ride — we created a strong bond. We wondered how things would change after having a child.

Father: From the very start, we included our son in our runs in a running stroller and later in cross country skiing outings in a backpack. The focus of my activities changed. I don't compete as much as just participate. I still enjoy the same rewards of setting and achieving goals. I got more gratification pushing a running stroller in a race than when, in the past, I used to cross the finish line ahead of others in my age group. The joy is greater because now my kids and I can share the pleasure of physical activity together.

When my son was almost two, I took him hiking up a mountain. It was only a twenty-minute hike for an adult, but we took about an hour. I could tell by the look on his face and his little swagger as we broke out of the woods at the top, that he too was starting to sense the pleasure we all get from exerting ourselves and achieving a goal. Since then, we have enjoyed many shared experiences like that. My children are now involved in competitive school sports. I have coached my son's travel soccer team for the past three years. This is a gratifying way to encourage and guide young athletes both on and off the field. Being a coach and "Dad" has provided time with my son and given us a chance to spend time together.

Mother: When our son was four weeks old, we hiked up a mountain carrying him in a front carrier. The view at the top was spectacular, but my eyes kept focusing on the small body sleeping in my arms. For me, parenthood changed my views on a lot of things in life. Fitness is one example. Staying healthy and fit, and sometimes competitive, is important — but not as important as raising healthy and happy children. Just as pregnancy was an opportunity to maintain a balance between exercise, diet, and rest, raising a health-oriented family is an outgrowth of those same goals. As I watch our son and daughter grow and change, it becomes increasingly apparent that so much of what they learn is based on what they see us, their parents, do. Perhaps waiting until age forty to start a family, working full time, and never having enough time, helped me set priorities. Now, as I enter "mid-life" my fitness routines have changed along with my families' activities. I no longer run competitively but savor my daily runs as a way to spend time alone and self reflect. My yoga practice has sustained me through the challenges of parenting and enabled me to maintain strength and flexibility. I am continuously finding ways to "fit in" my fitness. I am delighted like to see our son and daughter enjoy the sheer fun of physical activity, whether it is recreational or sport-oriented. I realize that that they are both gaining self-confidence, self-discipline, trust in their own bodies, and physical potential — all traits that will serve them well as they grow into adults.

"I've learned that you don't need to do 'mega' miles in running to stay in shape. More miles is not necessarily better." A triathlete

Reference List

American College of Obstetricians and Gynecologists (ACOG). *Exercise during Pregnancy and the Postpartum Period*. ACOG Committee Opinion, number 267, January 2002.

American College of Obstetricians and Gynecologists (ACOG). *Exercising During Pregnancy*. Educational pamphlet AP119. ACOG, Washington, D.C., June 2003.

American College of Sports Medicine. *ACSM's guidelines for exercise testing and prescription*. 6th ed. Philadelphia: Lippincott, Williams and Wilkins, 2000.

Anon. All About Children's Ski Sleds. www.xcskiworld.com/family/parents/sleds.

Anon. www.ibike.org/education/infant.htm.

Artal, R., & O'Toole, M. Guidelines of the American College of Obstetricians and Gynecologists for exercise during pregnancy and the postpartum period. *British Journal of Sports Medicine, 37,* 6-12. 2003.

Artal, R, Clapp, J. F., Vigil, D. Exercise during Pregnancy, *ACSM Current Comment*, August, 2000.

Artal, Raul. Exercise during Pregnancy. *The Physician and Sportsmedicine*, volume 27, number 8, August 1999.

Barrett, Jennifer and Teri Hanson, Yoga for Pregnancy and Beyond. *Fit Pregnancy*, January 2005.

Bell, R. J., Palma, S. M., & Lumley, J. M. The effect of vigorous exercise during pregnancy on birth-weight. *Australian Journal of Obstetrics and Gynaecology, 1,* 46-51, 1995.

Berk, Bonnie. Exercising on a Fitness Ball. www.pregnancyandbaby.com.

Brown, W. The benefits of physical activity during pregnancy. *Journal of Science and Medicine in Sport, 5*(1), 37-45, 2002.

Camporesi EM. Diving and pregnancy. *Semin Perinatol,* 20(4):292–302, 1996.

CDC. *Prevalence of overweight among children and adolescents*: United States, 1999--2002. National Health and Nutrition Examination Survey. Hyattsville, MD: US Department of Health and Human Services, CDC, National Center for Health Statistics. http://www.cdc.gov/nchs/products/pubs/pubd/hestats/overwght99.htm.

Clapp, James F. III. *Exercising Through Your Pregnancy*. Omaha: Addicus Books, 2002

Clapp, J. F., III. Recommending Exercise during Pregnancy. *Contemporary Ob/Gyn,* January 2001, pages 30-49.

Clapp, J. F., Little, K. D., & Capeless, E. L. Fetal heart rate response to sustained recreational exercise. *American Journal of Obstetrics and Gynecology, 168,*198-206, 1993.

Davies, G. A. L., Wolfe, L. A., Mottola, M. F., & MacKinnon, C. Joint SOGC/CSEP clinical practice guideline: Exercise in pregnancy and the postpartum period. *Canadian Journal of Applied Physiology, 28,* 329-341, 2003.

Dempsey, F C.; Butler, F L.; Williams, F A. No Need for a Pregnant Pause: Physical Activity May Reduce the Occurrence of Gestational Diabetes Mellitus and Preeclampsia. *Exercise & Sport Sciences Reviews*. 33(3):141-149, July 2005.

Evenson, K.R., et al. Vigorous Leisure Activity and Pregnancy Outcome. *Epidemiology,* volume 13, number 6, November 2002, pages 653-659.

Garshasbi A, Faghih Zadeh S. The effect of exercise on the intensity of low back pain in pregnant women. *Int J Gynaecol Obstet*. 88(3):271-5. March 2005.

Granatha, A., Hellgrenb, M, & Gunnarssonc,R Water Aerobics Reduces Sick Leave due to Low Back Pain During Pregnancy *Journal of Obstetric, Gynecologic, & Neonatal Nursing,* volume 35 page 465. July/August 2006

Hale, R.W., Milne L. The elite athlete and exercise in pregnancy. *Semin Perinatol* 1996.20:277-284

Hatch, M. C., Shu, X., McLean, D. E., Levin, B., Begg, M., Reus, L., et al. Maternal exercise during pregnancy, physical fitness, and fetal growth. *American Journal of Epidemiology, 137,* 1105-1114, 1993.

Huch, R. Physical activity at altitude in pregnancy. *SeminPerinatol,* 20(4):303–14, 1996.

Kardel, K. R., & Kase, T. Training in pregnant women: Effects on fetal development and birth. *American Journal of Obstetrics and Gynecology, 178,* 280-286, 1998.

Kardel,KR. Effects of intense training during and after pregnancy in top-level athletes. *Scand J Med Sci Sports.* Vol 2, April 2005, pages 67-8.

Katz VL. Water exercise in pregnancy. *Semin Perinatol* 1996;20(4):285–91.

Leet, T. & Flick, L. Effect of exercise on birthweight. *Clinical Obstetrics and Gynecology, 46,* 423-431, 2003.

Lumbers, E. R. Exercise in pregnancy: Physiological basis of exercise prescription for the pregnant woman. *Journal of Science and Medicine in Sport, 5*(1), 20-31, 2002.

Mittelmark, R. A., Wiswell, R. A., & Drinkwater, B. L. (Eds.) *Exercise in Pregnancy* (2nd ed). Baltimore: Williams & Wilkins, 1991.

Mottola MF. Exercise in the postpartum period: Practical applications. *Curr Sports Med* 2002;1:362–8.

Moyer-Mileur, Laurie. Why Prenatal Yoga Is So Popular. www.babycenter.com. June 2005.

O'Toole, M. L. Physiologic aspects of exercise in pregnancy. *Clinical Obstetrics and Gynecology, 46,* 379-389, 2003.

Paisley TS, Joy EA, Price RJ. Exercise during pregnancy: A practical approach. *Curr Sports Med Rep* 2003; 2:325–30.

Poudevigne and O'Connor. Physical activity and mood during pregnancy. *Med Sci Sports Exercise,* August 2005, pages 1374-80.

Rafla NM, Cook JR. The effect of maternal exercise on fetal heart rate. *J Obstet Gynaecol.* 1999 Jul;19(4):381-4.

Royal College of Obstetricians and Gynaecologists. Exercise in Pregnancy, Jan 2006.

Sampselle, C.M., et al. Physical Activity and Postpartum Well-Being. *Journal of Obstetric, Gynecologic and Neonatal Nursing,* January/February 1999, pages 41-49.

Selby, Anna. *Pilates for Pregnancy: Gentle and Effective Techniques for Before and After Birth.* Thorsons, 2002.

Sorgen, Carol. Having a Baby? Think Yoga? http://www.webmd.com/ February 2005.

Synder and Pendergraph. Exercise During Pregnancy: what do we really know? *American Family Physician*, March 1, 2004.

Sternfeld, B., Quesenberry, C. P., Eskenazi, B., & Newman, L. A. Exercise during pregnancy and pregnancy outcome. *Medicine and Science in Sports and Exercise, 27, 634-640,* 1995.

Troiano RP, Flegal KM, Kuczmarski RJ, Campbell SM, Johnson CL. Overweight prevalence and trends for children and adolescents. *Arch Pediatr Adolesc Med,* 149:1085-91, 1995.

U.S. Department of Health & Human Services. *Pregnancy and a Healthy Diet.* Washington, D.C., 2005.

Waehner, Paige. Pilates and Pregnancy: The Perfect Preparation for Labor and Delivery. www.pregnancytoday.com.

Resource Section

These are examples of resources available. A web search under a chosen topic will yield many more options for you.

Books

Adamany, Karrie *Post-Pregnancy Pilates An Essential Guide for a Fit Body After Baby,* Avery, 2005

Clapp, James F. III *Exercising Through Your Pregnancy,* Addicus Books, 2002

Cram, Catherine; Drenth ,Tere Stouffer *Fit Pregnancy for Dummies,* Wiley Publishing, 2004

Curtis, Glade B.; Schuler Judith *Your Pregnancy Quick Guide to Nutrition and Weight Management,* Da Capo Press, 2004

Fleming, Sue *Buff Moms-to-Be : The Complete Guide to Fitness for Expectant Mothers,* Villard, 2003

Gallo, Birgitta; Ross, Sheryl *Expecting Fitness : How To Modify And Enjoy Your Exercise Program Throughout Your Pregnancy,* Renaissance Books, 2000

Graves, Ginny *Pregnancy Fitness : Mind Body Spirit,* Three Rivers Press, 1999

Katz, Jane   *Water Fitness During Your Pregnancy*, Human Kinetics Publishers, 1995

King, Michael King; Green, Yolande *Pilates for Pregnancy,* Ulysses Press, 2002

Lundgren, Chris *Runner's World Guide to Running & Pregnancy,* Rodale Books, 2003

Nordahl, Karen; Petersen, Carl; Jeffreys, Renne Minges   *Fit to Deliver: An Innovative Prenatal and Postpartum Fitness Program*, Hartley & Marks Publishers, 2005

Selby, Anna *Pilates for Pregnancy: Gentle and Effective Techniques for Before and After Birth*, Thorsons, 2002

Teasdill, Wendy *Step-By-Step Yoga For Pregnancy: Essential Exercises for the Childbearing Year,* McGraw-Hill, 2000

Weiss, Robin Elise *The Everything Pregnancy Fitness Book* ,Adams Media Corporation, 2004

Winsor, Mari; Laska ,Mark *The Pilates Pregnancy: Maintaining Strength, Flexibility and Your Figure* Perseus, Publishing, 2001

Video

Erick, Miriam *Morning Sickness: All Day & All Night* Barrett Publishing Co.

DVDs

Pilates in Pregnancy Quantum Leap, 2004

Pregnancy Workout by Jazzercise

Rea, Shiva *Prenatal Yoga* Living Arts, 2000

Yoga for Your Pregnancy Good Times Video, 2004

Maternity Supplies – General

Baby Center Store   http://store.babycenter.com

Clothing

The following places offer affordable and comfortable maternity workout wear:

Mothers In Motion   www.mothersinmotion.com
Annacris.com   www.annacris.com
Fit Maternity   http://www.fitmaternity.com/
GapMaternity   www.gapmaternity.com

Equipment

(Note that some manufacturers make products that offer conversion kits so that a piece of equipment can serve more than one sport. The Chariot, for example, uses an enclosed carrier for the child and sells the bike, running, and ski attachments separately.)

► *Bicycles For Women*

Luna Cycles (custom)
218 Sombrio Drive
Santa Fe, NM 87501
http://www.lunacycles.com/index.html
505-231-0212

R+E Cycles (custom)
5627 University Way NE
Seattle, WA 98105
http://www.rodcycle.com/

Terry Precision Cycling
1657 East Park Drive
Macedon NY 14502
www.terrybicycles.com
800 289 8379

► *Bike Trailers*

Baby Jogger	www.babyjogger.com
Burley	www.burley.com
Chariot	www.chariotcarriers.com
InSTEP	www.instep.net
Schwinn	www.schwinnbike.com

► *Packs*

Baby Jogger	www.babyjogger.com
Baby Trend	www.babytrend.com
Deuter	www.deuterusa.com
Kelty	www.kelty.com
Tough Traveler	www.toughtraveler.com

▶ *Pulks (ski sleds)*

Baby Glider   www.babyglider.com
Chariot   www.chariotcarriers.com
Kifaru Sleds   www.kifaru.net/sleds (previously Mountainsmith Sleds)
Wilderness Engineering   www.wildernessengineering.com

▶ *Running Strollers*

Baby Trend   www.babytrend.com
Burley   www.burley.com
Chariot   www.chariotcarriers.com
InSTEP   www.instep.net
Kelty   `   www.kelty.com
Schwinn   www.schwinnbike.com

Organizations

American Academy of Pediatrics
141 Northwest Point Blvd
Elk Grove Village, IL 60007-1098
http://www.aap.org/
847-434-4000

American College of Nurse-Midwives
8403 Colesville Rd, Suite 1550
Silver Spring MD 20910
www.midwife.org
240-485-1800

American College of Obstetricians and Gynecologists
409 12th St., S.W., PO Box 96920
Washington, D.C. 20090-6920
(202) 638-5577
www.acog.org

American College of Sports Medicine
P.O. Box 1440
Indianapolis, IN 46206-1440
http://www.acsm.org
(317) 637-9200

American Council on Exercise
4851 Paramount Drive
San Diego, California 92123
http://www.acefitness.org/
1-800-825-3636

American Pregnancy Association
1425 Greenway Drive, Suite 440
Irving, Texas 75038
http://www.americanpregnancy.org/

March of Dimes
1275 Mamaroneck Avenue
White Plains, NY 10605
http://www.marchofdimes.com/

National Strength and Conditioning Association
1885 Bob Johnson Drive
Colorado Springs, CO 80906
http://nsca-lift.org/
719-632-6722

The National Women's Health Information Center
U.S. Department of Health ad Human Services
www.4women.gov
1-800-994-9662

Help and Support groups

La Leche League International -- a group that help mothers worldwide to breastfeed through mother-to-mother support, encouragement, information, and education and to promote a better understanding of breastfeeding as an important element in the healthy development of the baby and mother.   http://www.lalecheleague.org/ 1-800-laleche

Postpartum Support International -- a worldwide support group.
http://www.postpartum.net/

Sidelines -- a non-profit organization providing international support for women and their families experiencing complicated pregnancies and premature births.
http://www.sidelines.org/

Index